evidence
for nursing practice

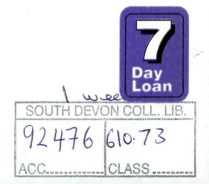

evidence
for nursing practice

MARY COURTNEY RN, PhD

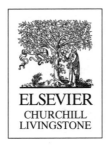

ELSEVIER
CHURCHILL
LIVINGSTONE

Sydney   Edinburgh   London   New York   Philadelphia   St Louis   Toronto

ELSEVIER

Churchill Livingstone
is an imprint of Elsevier

Elsevier Australia
30–52 Smidmore Street, Marrickville, NSW 2204

This edition © 2005 Elsevier Australia
(a division of Reed International Books Australia Pty Ltd)
ACN 001 002 357

National Library of Australia Cataloguing-in-Publication Data

---

Courtney, Mary D. (Mary Denise).
 Evidence for nursing practice.

Includes index.
For tertiary students.
 ISBN 0 7295 3744 7.

1. Evidence-based nursing. 2. Nursing – Decision making.
I. Title.

610.73

Publisher: Vaughn Curtis
Publishing editor: Mary Maakaroun
Publishing services manager: Helena Klijn
Project coordinator: Emma Hutchinson
Editor and project manager: Ruth Matheson
Cover and internal designer: Design Animals
Typesetter: Sun Photoset Pty Ltd
Proofreader: Pam Dunne
Indexer: Max McMaster
Printed and bound in Australia by Ligare

contents ─────────────●

Part 1 Introduction

1 Evidence-based nursing practice 3
Mary Courtney, Claire Rickard, Joy Vickerstaff and Anthea Court

Part 2 How to search for current best evidence

2 Using the right type of evidence to answer clinical questions 37
Joan Webster and Sonya Osborne

7   Assessing the effectiveness of screening and diagnostic tests 103
Wendy Chaboyer and Lukman Thalib

8   Outcomes for evidence-based nursing practice 115
Anne Chang

Part 4 Implementing evidence in practice

9   Developing a culture of inquiry to sustain evidence-based practice . . 135
Sonya Osborne and Glenn Gardner

Part 5 Measurement of nursing health outcomes

13 Instruments for measuring symptoms 201
Patsy Yates

14 Instruments to measure health-related quality of life as a nursing outcome 214
Jan McDowell and Helen Edwards

preface

Over the last decade, the Australian healthcare system has increasingly come under siege to improve the quality and access of patient care within a context of increasingly limited resources. Greater emphasis is being placed on all health professionals to seek out best practice evidence and apply it in their everyday practice.

As there are large gaps in the amount of robust evidence for much of what nurses do during the course of their daily work, the challenge for nurses is to develop and implement well-focused evidence-based nursing interventions and treatments in order to improve the quality of patient care.

This book will create a text that provides a step-by-step guide for both experienced registered nurses and students of nursing on how to find, appraise and use appropriate evidence in their everyday practice.

This text is divided into five parts:

1. Part 1 examines what evidence-based practice (EBP) is. It introduces the reader to the development of the EBP movement and provides an overview of why EBP has spread so rapidly over the last decade. It outlines strategies for incorporating evidence into practice, while overviewing education, research and practice challenges for the future.
2. Part 2 focuses on how to search for current best evidence. It details types of evidence, and examines both quantitative and qualitative research designs to gather evidence. It concludes with a chapter on how to undertake a systematic review.
3. Part 3 examines how to critically appraise the evidence. The three chapters in this section examine: the effectiveness of nursing interventions; the effectiveness of diagnostic tests and screening; and the validity of nursing and health outcomes evidence.
4. Part 4 focuses on how to implement evidence in practice. This section provides four chapters on: developing an evidence-based culture; undertaking an audit; undertaking a program evaluation; and developing evidence-based guidelines.
5. Part 5 examines 'how' instruments are used for measuring nursing and health outcomes, and focuses on pain and symptom management, as well as quality of life, functional assessment and psychosocial aspects of health.

A range of discussion points and case studies are included to assist readers using this book as a text.

If you find any errors as you read through this book, please let me know. I will acknowledge your good detective work when the book is printed again. Also, any feedback you may have that might assist in the refinement of subsequent editions of this text would be gratefully appreciated.

Finally, many thanks to all the contributing authors for providing the expertise and experience required to draw together the material for the complex issues and practices addressed in this book.

Mary Courtney

contributors ●

Editor

Courtney, Mary RN, PhD is Professor of Nursing and Director of Research, School of Nursing, Queensland University of Technology, and Honorary Research Consultant, Royal Brisbane and Women's Hospital Health Service District

Chapter authors

Battistutta, Diana BSc (Hons), PhD is Lecturer in Biostatistics, School of Public Health, Queensland University of Technology

Borbasi, Sally RN, PhD, Associate Professor, School of Nursing and Midwifery, Flinders University, South Australia

Chaboyer, Wendy RN, PhD is Professor of Nursing and Director, Research Centre for Clinical Practice Innovation, Griffith University, Gold Coast, Queensland

Chang, Anne RN, PhD is Director, Joanna Briggs Institute, Mater Hospital, Brisbane, and Professor of Nursing, School of Nursing, Queensland University of Technology

Court, Anthea is Associate Director—Evidence Transfer & Utilisation, Joanna Briggs Institute, Department of Clinical Nursing, University of Adelaide

Duggan, Geraint is Project Manager, National Institute of Clinical Studies (NICS), Melbourne

Edwards, Helen RN, PhD is Professor of Nursing and Head, School of Nursing, Queensland University of Technology

Field, John RN, BLegSt, ADNE, GradCertManag is Senior Lecturer and Director, International Programs and Strategic Alliances, School of Nursing and Midwifery, La Trobe University, Melbourne

FitzGerald, Mary RN, PhD is Professor of Nursing, University of Newcastle, NSW, and Central Coast Health

Gardner, Glenn RN, PhD is Director, Centre for Clinical Nursing, Royal Brisbane and Women's Hospital Health Service District and Professor of Clinical Nursing, School of Nursing, Queensland University of Technology

Jackson, Debra RN, PhD is Associate Professor, School of Nursing, Family and Community Health, College of Social and Health Sciences, University of Western Sydney

Lockwood, Craig RN, BN, GradDipClinNurs, MNSc is Deputy Director, Centre for Evidence-based Nursing, South Australia, Royal Adelaide Hospital, and Clinical Tutor, Department of Clinical Nursing, University of Adelaide

Manias, Elizabeth RN, PhD is Associate Professor, School of Nursing, University of Melbourne

McDowell, Jan RN, PhD is Senior Research Fellow, and Lee Foundation Fellow in Diabetes Research, Centre for Health Research (Nursing), Queensland University of Technology

Osborne, Sonya RN, BSN, MN is Nurse Researcher, Centre for Clinical Nursing, Royal Brisbane and Women's Hospital Health Service District

Pearson, Alan RN, PhD is National Director, Joanna Briggs Institute, Adelaide University, South Australia, and Professor of Nursing, La Trobe University, Melbourne

Rickard, Claire RN, PhD is Lecturer, Centre for Multidisciplinary Studies in Rural Health, Monash University

Thalib, Lukman BSc (Hons, Biometry), MSc (Biometry), PhD is a Medical Statistician and Assistant Professor in the Faculty of Medicine at Kuwait University, Kuwait

Vickerstaff, Joy RN, BA, MCogSci is National Institute of Clinical Studies (NICS) Board Director and Executive Director of Nursing Services, Princess Alexandra Hospital and District Health Service, Queensland, and Adjunct Associate Professor, Queensland University of Technology

Webster, Joan RN, BA is Nursing Director, Research, Royal Brisbane and Women's Hospital Health Service District, and Adjunct Associate Professor, Queensland University of Technology

Yates, Patsy RN, PhD is Professor and Acting Director of the Centre for Palliative Care Research and Education, Queensland University of Technology

part one

Introduction

chapter ①

Evidence-based nursing practice

Mary Courtney, Claire Rickard, Joy Vickerstaff and Anthea Court

1.1 Learning objectives

After reading this chapter, you should be able to:

1. *understand what is evidence-based practice (EBP)*
2. *understand the benefits and alternatives to using EBP*
3. *explain what has caused the major spread of the EBP movement*
4. *list where evidence may be located to support best practice*
5. *describe two major structures promoting the utilisation of EBP in Australia—the National Institute for Clinical Studies (NICS) and the Joanna Briggs Institute (JBI)*
6. *explain how evidence may be incorporated into nursing practice, and*
7. *discuss the challenges the EBP-based movement has posed for both nursing education and nursing research.*

1.2 Introduction

This chapter introduces the reader to the development of the EBP movement and provides an overview of why EBP has spread so rapidly over the last decade. It explains how evidence may be incorporated into nursing practice and examines the challenges the EBP-based movement has posed for both nursing education and nursing research.

1.3 What is 'evidence-based practice'?

Health professionals currently advise their patients to stop smoking. Why do they give this advice? Why don't they advise them to start smoking or increase their smoking intake? The reason is that evidence is available that demonstrates:

- high levels of smoking are associated with increased risk of lung cancer, and
- stopping smoking reduces the risk of lung cancer.

This is an example of evidence that can identify the cause of a disease and the effectiveness of an intervention to improve patient outcomes and decrease illness and disability.

The development of EBP can be traced back to the work of a group of researchers at MacMaster University in Ontario, Canada, who set out to redefine the practice of medicine to improve the usability of information (Lockett 1997).

The term 'evidence-based practice' or EBP has been derived from the earlier work of evidence-based medicine. Earlier years saw the development of EBP practice limited to the discourse of 'medicine'; however, more recently many other health professional groups have moved to use EBP principles in their practice—for example, orthodontics (Harrison 2000) and allied health therapies (Bury & Mead 1998).

In 1997, Sackett et al (1997:2) published the first textbook on evidence-based medicine and defined it as:

> The conscientious, explicit and judicious use of current best
> evidence in making decisions about the healthcare of patients.

In 2000, Sackett et al (2000) also included patient values as well as clinical expertise:

> The practice . . . integrates clinical expertise and patient values
> with the best available research evidence.

Critics of EBP have described it as 'cookbook' healthcare, or the worship of science above human experience. However, these criticisms are easily defused by an understanding of the three-factor interaction that EBP promotes: the best available research evidence; clinical expertise; and patient values (see Fig 1.1).

Figure 1.1 The three elements of evidence-based practice

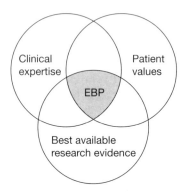

Source: Sackett et al 2000.

JAMA, the *Journal of the American Medical Association*, has been committed to publishing 'Users' guides' to the research literature, with an excellent series of 25 articles on the topic published from 1993 to 2000. An important resource is a compendium of these articles, with further commentary, published in book form in 2002 (Guyatt & Rennie 2002). Although the guides are aimed primarily at a medical audience, they are highly appropriate for all health practitioners, including not only traditional quantitative/epidemiological approaches but also guides to interpreting qualitative evidence for practice (Giacomini 2000a, 2000b).

Therefore, EBP is not only applying research-based evidence to assist in making decisions about the healthcare of patients, but rather extends to identifying knowledge gaps, finding and systematically appraising and condensing the evidence to assist clinical expertise, rather than replace it (Tarling & Crofts 1998:24).

1.4 What are the benefits of evidence-based practice?

There are benefits of EBP to: patients/consumers; nurses; the healthcare organisation; and the community.

1.4.1 To patients/consumers

To healthcare consumers, it may seem ludicrous, or even frightening, that the EBP concept is relatively new. Patients typically accept recommended care from health professionals with the unspoken assumption that the practitioner knows what works.

1.4.2 To nurses

In an ideal world, nurses could keep up to date by reading all of the published literature in their relevant area. In reality, with approximately a thousand new publications each year relevant to surgical nursing for example, this is clearly an impossible task. EBP allows a more structured and streamlined way of keeping abreast of relevant new developments without becoming overwhelmed by information overload.

EBP also allows nurses to communicate effectively with their patients and with the healthcare team about the rationales for decision making and care plans. An EBP nurse is a confident professional, feeling assured that they are providing care that is supported by facts rather than habits, and can take legal accountability for their practice.

1.4.3 To the healthcare organisation

Commitment to EBP philosophy allows healthcare organisations to position themselves in the market as quality institutions. An EBP-compliant institution should be less likely to attract litigation, or to successfully defend the care delivered, if it was in line with international best evidence at the time of care. In addition, EBP allows the scrutinising of practice for effectiveness. This process often results in practice changes that allow significant cost savings, or alternatively justify necessary additional expenditure. This is attractive to organisations frequently struggling to meet assigned budgetary limits, or lobbying government for additional funds.

1.4.4 To the community

Through the utilisation of EBP, finite resources are not wasted on the delivery of ineffective interventions. Additionally, EBP limits the amount of disability and suffering throughout the community by ensuring the most current and effective care is provided.

1.5 What are the alternatives to evidence-based practice?

You may be wondering how nurses made decisions about their practice before the relatively recent EBP movement, or even what are the alternatives to EBP. If we are honest, for most of our working life, we function on 'automatic pilot'—that is, we ritualistically do things the way we have always done them, the way we were taught as a student or graduate nurse, or just in the 'accepted' way of doing things in our current workplace.

However, at times our comfort zone is challenged, and we identify a knowledge deficit when confronting an unusual or challenging problem. At times like these, practitioners may guide their practice by asking the opinion of colleagues or senior practitioners, reviewing employer policies, reading textbooks or lecture notes, leafing through nursing or other journals, and listening to speakers at professional conferences or other education forums. Can you think of some benefits and limitations to these methods of guiding practice? For example, if a decision needs to be made immediately, guidance from an experienced colleague or organisational manual provides a quick and easy reference tool. However, on the downside, even well-meaning and senior practitioners may not have the latest knowledge, and policy manuals are frequently out-of-date, even if they were prepared using the best evidence at the time of policy development.

1.6 Why the rapid spread of evidence-based practice?

Some of the major reasons cited by Sackett et al (1997) for the spread of the EBP movement have been:
- the lack of research-based information to support clinical decision making
- the lack of research-based guidelines and protocols to use in clinical practice
- the overwhelming volume and variability of new journal information, and
- the inadequacy of traditional sources of information (e.g. textbooks out-of-date).

However, health departments around the world are increasingly being stretched to cover ever-rising health expenditures and, with treatment and care costs increasing all the time, governments need to ensure they are using public funds for treatment and care that is effective with positive health outcomes and benefits for the public.

While it may be commendable to take the view that health departments have encouraged the development of EBP because they genuinely wish for patients to receive the best available care and to have the fewest adverse events as possible, unfortunately, the reality may more likely be that ineffective care and adverse events are very costly in terms of extended lengths of stay in expensive hospital beds and require additional costs such as pharmaceuticals, pathology tests and radiography. Additionally, poor patient care and mistakes also lead to threats of litigation (Tarling & Crofts 1998).

While EBP was initially limited to the practice of medicine it became clear that unless all the members of the health team embraced EBP it would have limited impact.

1.7 Where is the evidence located?

Evidence for practice decisions is increasingly available in online format. Some resources are available free of charge, while others attract a fee-for-use, although staff and students of healthcare facilities and universities can usually access these through the institution at no personal cost. New products are constantly being developed to allow practitioners to quickly and easily search for relevant evidence; however, some of the currently well-established and recommended sources of evidence are described below.

1.7.1 CINAHL®

The CINAHL® (Cumulative Index to Nursing and the Allied Health Literature) database covers the nursing, allied health and health sciences literature from 1982 to the present. Originally a printed index, the CINAHL database has been available as a web-based product since 1994. CINAHL includes 3.6 million citations in the database and is growing weekly. Most citations have abstracts and some are provided as full-text articles. Individuals can subscribe to CINAHL for a fee; however, as most health facilities and universities are subscribers, access is available free to their staff and students. Contact your librarian to find out whether your institution has CINAHL access. See www.cinahl.com/.

1.7.2 Medline

Medline is compiled by the US National Library of Medicine and is acknowledged as the world's most comprehensive source of bibliographic information for health. Medline includes literature from the nursing, medicine and allied health disciplines, as well as the health humanities, and dentistry, veterinary, biological, physical and information science. Medline has nearly 11 million records dating from 1965 to the present and is updated weekly. Subscription through various commercial platforms is available for a fee to both individuals and institutions, and is widely available for free to staff and students of subscribing health facilities and universities. Medline is also available free of charge from any computer connected to the internet through a package called Pubmed. See www.ncbi.nlm.nih.gov/PubMed/.

1.7.3 The Cochrane Library

An important resource for EBP is the Cochrane Library, which is produced by the international Cochrane Collaboration. Material included has been pre-filtered for quality of evidence and clinical applicability, and is updated quarterly. The Library consists of several databases.

The Cochrane Database of Systematic Reviews (CDSR) was launched in 2000 and includes over 3500 full-text systematic reviews of high-quality research undertaken by Cochrane collaborators that are designed to answer specific clinical questions. The Database of Abstracts of Reviews of Effects (DARE) includes over 4500 structured abstracts of systematic reviews undertaken outside the Cochrane Collaboration. The Cochrane Central Register of Controlled Trials (CENTRAL) includes details of over 400,000 controlled trials published in journals as well as reports from conference proceedings and other sources not currently listed in other bibliographic databases.

Other materials include the Cochrane Methodology Register (CMR), the National Health Service Economic Evaluation Database (NHSEED) and the Health Technology Assessment (HTA) database. All residents of Australia can access the Cochrane Library for free online due to funding provided by the Commonwealth Government and administered by the National Institute of Clinical Studies (NICS). See www.nicsl.com.au/cochrane/index.asp.

1.7.4 PsycINFO

The PsycINFO database is the premier online collection of bibliographic references covering the psychological literature from 1872 to the present, including articles from over 1300 journals. Most references include abstracts or content summaries. In addition to journal articles, many books, chapters and academic dissertations are included. PsycINFO is a fee-for-product service that is widely available at no charge to practitioners through subscribing health libraries. See www.psycinfo.com/psycinfo/.

1.7.5 Meditext

Meditext was launched in 2001 and contains material from the Australian Medical Index (AMI) compiled by the National Library of Australia. Indexed are over 160 Australian and New Zealand health journals and other materials such as conference proceedings and government reports. Many Meditext references are materials not included in Medline. Some full-text documents and links to full-text articles are included. The majority of universities and health departments provide fee-free access to their staff and students. See www.copyright.com.au/online_projects_meditext.htm.

1.7.6 The 'grey' literature

The 'grey' literature is a term used to refer to evidence that exists in some format but is difficult to find due to its non-inclusion in searchable bibliographic indexes such as Medline, which predominantly contain references to articles in highly ranked peer-refereed journals. While some grey literature may not be contained in such journals because it is of poor quality, this is not always the case, and a thorough literature search will also make efforts to identify relevant research that may have been published only in conference proceedings, non-refereed journals, government/organisational reports, textbooks or the popular press, as well as academic theses that may or may not have been followed up with publication. Some efforts have been made to assist clinicians to search or access the grey literature including aspects of the Cochrane Collaboration (see Section 1.7.3) and the following online instruments: the Australian Digital Theses (ADT) Program and the Conference Papers Index.

1.7.6.1 The Australian Digital Theses (ADT) Program

The ADT Program began in 1998, and has been open to all Australian universities since 2000. It consists of a national collaborative of digitised theses produced at Australian universities (PhD and Masters by Research theses only). The program can be accessed free of charge via any internet-connected computer. See http://adt.caul.edu.au/.

1.7.6.2 The Conference Papers Index

This database provides over 1.5 million citations to oral papers and poster sessions presented at major scientific conferences internationally from 1982 to the present. Major areas of subject coverage include healthcare, as well as biochemistry, chemistry, biology, biotechnology and many others. The Index is updated bimonthly and is available through subscribing health or academic institutions. See www.csa.com/csa/factsheets/cpilong.shtml.

1.8 Major structures promoting evidence-based practice

In Australia and New Zealand, the major structures promoting EBP are: the National Institute of Clinical Studies (NICS); the Joanna Briggs Institute (JBI); the Centre for Evidence Based Nursing—Aotearoa (CEBNA); and the New Zealand Guidelines Group.

1.8.1 The National Institute of Clinical Studies (NICS)

Reliable data on the gaps between clinical evidence (what research shows that clinicians should be doing in their clinical care) and clinical practice (what is actually done) is often difficult to find. Despite this there have been sufficient published research studies to suggest that there is a gaps problem in many healthcare systems. Dutch and American studies indicate that between 30% and 40% of patients do not receive care based on best research evidence, and that 20–25% of the care provided is either not needed or may be potentially harmful (Schuster et al 1988, Grol 2001).

The National Institute of Clinical Studies (NICS) is Australia's national agency for improving healthcare by helping to close the gaps between best available evidence and current clinical practice. It was established as an Australian Government-owned company, run by a board of directors directly appointed by the Minister for Health, and commenced operations in 2001.

1.8.1.1 Why the need for the NICS?

In an editorial in the *Medical Journal of Australia* (Silagy 2001) the inaugural Chair of NICS, the late Chris Silagy, observed that the language and concepts of evidence-based healthcare have become institutionalised in most spheres of healthcare, yet there are still significant gaps between evidence and practice.

Silagy noted that since the inception of evidence-based medicine there has been considerable emphasis on what he termed 'upstream' strategies to support EBP, an emphasis characterised by huge numbers of systematic reviews, health technology assessments and clinical guidelines being made available to clinicians. This emphasis, however, had come without adequate consideration of the 'downstream' strategies necessary to ensure effective uptake and implementation of best evidence by clinicians. The mission of the NICS is to assist clinicians to turn this evidence into action.

1.8.1.2 What is important?

In planning a strategy to address the evidence–practice gaps in Australia one of the first tasks of the NICS was to work with clinicians in a series of consultation rounds to identify the gaps that are considered widespread, clinically significant and urgent. Professional colleges, societies, special interest groups and policy-making bodies were all invited to make submissions and the views of nurses, who make up over 70% of the Australian healthcare workforce, were particularly sought. The consultation process identified a number of clinical areas, including the care of patients treated in emergency departments and the care of patients with heart failure, as suboptimal when compared to best research evidence.

In 2002 the NICS established a nursing reference group of clinicians and academics to offer high-level advice on important practice gaps, and as a result of their recommendations the NICS began work to scope opportunities to close the gaps in pain management and pressure area management. This led to the NICS embarking on a major project to improve pain management in hospitalised patients with cancer, while the latter recommendation led the NICS to scope pressure area care in Australia. While this has not led to a major clinical project, because a number of other organisations are already working in this field, the NICS has been able to bring together a number of key Australian pressure area care resources in the NICS pressure ulcer resource guide (NICS website at www.nicsl.com.au).

Identification of EBP gaps is an evolutionary process and the NICS has recently published the first in a projected series of reports highlighting important gaps identified by doctors, nurses, allied health clinicians and policy makers in Australia (NICS 2003). As our understanding of what actually happens in clinical practice improves, through better integration of routine data-collection systems at the surgery and bedside, it is anticipated that many more clinically significant gaps will be identified in the coming years.

1.8.1.3 What do we know about what works?

The second task of the NICS was to bring together the disparate body of work on changing clinician behaviour into a coherent whole. Industries such as mining and aviation have approached behaviour change in a two-pronged way, from both a systemic and an individual perspective. While there is still an emphasis on individual responsibility, there has also been a corresponding reduction in the discretion of individuals to act autonomously, in favour of the introduction of industry-wide systems and protocols. This has resulted in significant improvements in safety. Attempts to change clinical behaviour in the healthcare industry have, to date, focused almost exclusively on the role of the individual clinician in areas such as supporting individual clinical decision making, and there have been very few initiatives that have looked at system-wide approaches to change. One important factor that has inhibited more widespread attempts at system-wide improvement is the lack of a sound scientific evidence base for the many strategies that have been proposed to date.

The NICS is in the process of using expertise from areas such as behavioural psychology and marketing to better identify ways of systematically changing clinician behaviour in Australia. An important part of this process will be to strengthen the evidence base of clinician behaviour strategies. Late in 2003 the NICS convened a national workshop of clinicians and policy makers with an expertise in change management to identify better ways to manage change in Australian healthcare; the results of the workshop have recently been published (NICS 2004).

1.8.1.4 Undertaking and studying change

The NICS clinical priority areas (described in Appendix 1.1) use specific change methods, such as plan–do–study–act (or 'breakthrough') collaboratives, academic detailing, focus groups, education packages, consumer education and internet-based strategies; each is designed to influence groups of clinicians and consumers in the most effective way. In adopting these methods the NICS subjects them to scientific evaluation in an attempt to identify what works in the Australian context, and what elements are transferable to other sectors of healthcare.

In one example the NICS ran Australia's first national collaborative, which targeted care in hospital emergency departments, using the plan–do–study–act methodology used by organisations such as the American Institute for Healthcare Improvement (Berwick 1998) and the British NHS Modernisation Agency (NHS website at www.modern.nhs.uk). What has become apparent is that while this method of quality improvement can be used successfully to make short-term health system changes, there has been little scientific research into the sustainability of such changes, and into the factors that determine whether, and how well, the method will work in particular settings.

While running its collaborative the NICS commissioned research using Change-Tracking® methodology to measure workplace culture before, during and after the collaborative, in an attempt to identify the relationship between workplace culture and capacity for clinical change. Similarly, another NICS-commissioned research project will involve a return to hospital emergency departments one year after the collaborative has finished, in an effort to better understand whether the short-term improvements noted during the collaborative can translate into embedded, system-wide changes in the longer term.

1.8.1.5 Clinical leaders

The third task of the NICS has been to foster clinical champions for change in Australia. In a series of programs that offer targeted grants, fellowships, scholarships and research funding in a variety of settings (described further in Appendix 1.1), the NICS hopes to identify and nurture clinicians in their early to mid-careers who, supported by NICS expertise in change management, will become Australia's next generation of clinical leaders.

These leaders face significant barriers. Implementation of research is still the poor relation of primary research and many clinicians face unique pressures as they try to implement change. Potential clinical leaders are often trapped by the competing requirements of teaching and clinical care, particularly in the context of severe workforce shortages, and it is hoped that the fellowship program in particular will allow clinicians 'space' to devote time and energy to developing large-scale implementation programs.

One important role the NICS is taking to support clinical leaders is to lobby research funders in Australia to commit a greater proportion of research grants to studies of implementation of primary research.

1.8.1.6 Working with others

The fourth task of the NICS is to develop tools to assist clinicians in implementing evidence-based healthcare. In 2002 the NICS acted on behalf of the Australian Government to purchase open access to the Cochrane Library, the best available source of appraised clinical evidence on the effects of intervention, for all Australian residents. Recognising the difficulty many clinicians and consumers face in navigating the library's interface, the NICS has worked with the Australasian Cochrane Centre to produce a comprehensive online users' guide to the library (see the Cochrane Centre website at www.nicsl.com.au/cochrane).

Other tools developed by the NICS for clinicians include a range of literature reviews on a number of diverse topics such as factors supporting high performance in healthcare organisations and the effectiveness of clinical information services, a scanning service where relevant journals and websites are regularly monitored, a database linking Australian-based clinical effectiveness researchers and the development of sophisticated web-based tools to support collaborative projects.

The NICS works closely with colleges, societies and organisations representing primary care, hospital medicine, nursing, allied health and indigenous health, as well as national and state-based organisations working in the areas of quality and safety, rural and remote care, guideline development and health insurance. It is only through close relationships with clinicians and policy makers at the clinical interface that the NICS is able to help close EBP gaps. The NICS will continue to build strong working alliances with both Australian and international organisations to improve healthcare.

Australia is not alone in recognising and addressing EBP gaps and strong relationships have been built with groups in New Zealand, Sweden, the United Kingdom, Canada, the United States and the Netherlands. The NICS has embarked on a long-term program inviting overseas experts to Australia to share their experiences and foster international dialogue on common problems. Despite workforce challenges and EBP gaps, most of the healthcare delivered in Australia is of a very high standard, and the NICS has a role in sharing Australian solutions, as well as seeking answers to local problems.

1.8.1.7 The future

The NICS continues to work in its chosen clinical priority areas and is embarking on a major initiative in the primary-care sector. Work continues on identifying the best and most suitable models to adopt to influence clinical practice change, and work will begin examining the three areas of clinical practice guidelines, clinical research implementation networks and communities of practice. The latter are networks established to increase and promote the sharing and use of information and problem solving in groups with a common interest, and have been used successfully in the information technology and engineering industries. In undertaking all this work the NICS is committed to publishing data that will clearly identify what has been tried and what works in specific Australian settings.

Nursing remains a crucial area of engagement for the NICS. As the numerically largest discipline that delivers most of the direct clinical care throughout all sectors of Australian healthcare, nurses are critical to the success of strategies to effectively close the gaps between evidence and practice. Nurses have been instrumental to the success of the work of the NICS in emergency care and will be central to the NICS strategy to improve the assessment and management of pain in hospitalised cancer patients. As the work of the NICS now moves into primary care and chronic disease management, it is ever-more important to identify, to understand and to disseminate nursing solutions throughout the Australian healthcare system.

1.8.2 The Joanna Briggs Institute (JBI)

The Joanna Briggs Institute (JBI) was established in 1996 and brings together a range of practice-oriented research activities to increase the effectiveness of healthcare practice and improvement of healthcare outcomes by:

- translating evidence (through systematic reviews of quantitative and qualitative research)
- transferring evidence (through such things as publications and workshops), and
- utilising evidence (through implementation projects and the Practical Application of Clinical Evidence System).

From its very small beginnings in 1996, the Institute is now a growing, dynamic international collaboration of over 400 researchers across 25 countries.

1.8.2.1 The Joanna Briggs Collaboration

The Joanna Briggs Collaboration is a coordinated effort by a group of self-governing collaborative centres, coordinated through the leadership of the JBI. The legitimate operations of the Joanna Briggs Collaboration include: the promotion of evidence-based healthcare; education and training; the conduct of systematic reviews; the development of *Best Practice* information sheets; the implementation of EBP; and the conduct of evaluation cycles and primary research arising out of systematic reviews.

Collaborating Centres are self-governing partners who accept the terms of the JBI Memorandum of Understanding. Centres are eligible to apply for grants funded through membership fees, but are expected to seek funds within their jurisdiction. Some Centres have a geographic jurisdiction, while others have a specialist jurisdiction. The Joanna Briggs Collaboration currently consists of 18 Collaborating Centres across the world. See Appendix 1.2 for a comprehensive list of these Centres.

In 1996 the first chair of the JBI management committee, Associate Professor Kaye Challinger, predicted that, 'the new institute would have a positive influence on nursing and healthcare delivery'. Now, the JBI and its Collaboration is having an impact on healthcare not just in Australasia, but also throughout the world. A broad membership base consisting primarily of healthcare and education facilities financially supports research conducted by the JBI. These members receive access to a variety of evidence-based information to inform clinical practice, journals and other publications of the JBI, as well as supporting the ongoing research activity of the JBI.

13

Much of the information produced by the JBI is available both electronically and in hard-copy format to assist in accessibility via varied access options. The JBI website (see www.joannabriggs.edu.au) has also proven to be a useful tool for both students and practising health professionals. To provide access to this best available evidence a number of the JBI's products are available on the website at no cost.

One of the core activities of the JBI is to translate and transfer research information relevant to clinical practice. The emerging systematic review methodology and emphasis of relevance to the clinical area has led to the development of software to assist in the conduct of *comprehensive systematic reviews*. SUMARI (System for the Unified Management of Assessment and Review Information) is in development to provide researchers with an online system that will enable creation of systematic reviews that consider all forms of research on a specific topic, including qualitative, narrative and opinion, economic data as well as quantitative papers. The inclusion of these areas is most appropriate for healthcare issues that cannot be measured by way of randomised controlled trial. The inclusion of qualitative research has also led to the consideration of Feasibility, Appropriateness and Meaningfulness of an intervention as well as simply the Effectiveness (i.e. the JBI-initiated FAME scale). This is discussed further in Chapter 6.

From systematic reviews the JBI develops *Best Practice* information sheets, a guideline series designed specifically to inform health professionals of the best available evidence. The first *Best Practice* information sheet was produced in September 1997 and distributed through nursing journals in Australia and New Zealand. In 2004, the *Best Practice* series continues to be distributed through journals, but it is now also distributed to members globally and translated into Italian and Japanese.

One of the challenges facing researchers who produce guidelines in the twenty-first century is that of utilisation. It has been recognised for some time that distributing evidence-based guidelines alone does not alter clinical practice and that change management strategies need to be employed to achieve and maintain valuable change (NHS Centres for Reviews and Dissemination 1999). Researchers at the JBI are taking up the challenge and developing the utilisation tool Practical Application of Clinical Evidence System (PACES). PACES is designed to assist healthcare facilities to audit practice, respond to results of audit and to change and evaluate this response. This program will also incorporate 'GRIP' (Getting Research Into Practice), to assist in the identification of priority areas for evidence utilisation, the examination of barriers, and the design and evaluation of implementation programs employed to overcome the identified barriers.

Evaluating the influence of the JBI-produced information on healthcare delivery is necessary to determine the benefit of continuing research of this type. The impact of the *Best Practice* series along with its recommendations has been evaluated by way of a survey conducted throughout Australia and New Zealand. Survey results indicate that of those who had read *Best Practice*, around 25% of first-survey respondents specifically altered their practice. This figure increased to over 35% in the second survey just three years later. Before-and-after-style multisite evaluations are also conducted to examine the effect of recommendations of *Best Practice* in the clinical setting.

Critical appraisal skills are also promoted and supported by the JBI. RAPid (Rapid Appraisal Protocol internet database) has been developed as a training program to organise, conduct and archive an evidence summary of the findings of a single study or systematic review. RAPid facilitates study-type recognition, data extraction and the construction of a final report, which may then be submitted online to the RAPid library for independent critique. Then, if it is accepted, it is uploaded for worldwide access. This program is uniquely suitable for use by university lecturers and facilitators of continuing education in health services for training and integration into curricula. RAPid may motivate students to become active in the publication of their work and to experience the benefits of disseminating knowledge to their profession.

It is anticipated that the products and services of the JBI will continue to develop and grow according to the changing needs of the healthcare profession. The staff of the JBI are committed to regularly examining the products and services offered, and to implementing change as required by members of the JBI.

1.8.3 The Centre for Evidence Based Nursing—Aotearoa (CEBNA)

The Centre for Evidence Based Nursing (CEBNA) is the predominant nursing organisation promoting EBP in New Zealand. It is a collaboration between the Auckland District Health Board and the University of Auckland, School of Nursing. CEBNA also partners with the JBI for evidence-based nursing and midwifery. The Centre's activities include the conduct of systematic reviews, research and research training. See www.health.auckland.ac.nz/cebna/.

1.8.4 The New Zealand Guidelines Group (NZGG)

The New Zealand Guidelines Group (NZGG) was established in 1996 by the National Health Committee (NHC) as an informal expert network on practice guideline development and implementation. Since 1999, NZGG has been an independent government-funded society with offices in Wellington and Auckland. Representatives from nursing, Maori Health, Pacific Health, consumer representation, medicine, disability support, public health medicine and general practice govern NZGG. The role of NZGG is to provide tools to promote an evidence-based culture within the New Zealand health and disability sector. Activities include production of evidence-based guidelines, distribution of evidence-based information from New Zealand and overseas, and training in guideline development and implementation. See www.nzgg.org.nz/.

1.9 How can evidence be incorporated into nursing practice?

There are a variety of situations in which nursing practice (and, therefore, nurses) draws on evidence bases. Nurses are not only limited to the medical science evidence, but also extend their EBP to the behavioural and social sciences. Some examples are outlined below.

1.9.1 Nursing care intervention evidence

Nurses make clinical decisions about interventions concerning investigations, observations or drugs, and therefore draw upon evidence from a range of different sources. For example, psychosocial evidence as well as pharmacological knowledge may be sought in instigating a particular nursing intervention, as may evidence on cost-effectiveness. Therefore, it is crucial that nurses understand the variety of perspectives of evidence when undertaking an intervention.

Case study: Should central venous line catheter administration sets be changed biweekly or left intact?

Modern healthcare involves many invasive diagnostic and treatment interventions. Additionally, many chronically or seriously ill patients who would once have had a poor prognosis can now expect an improved life span, although this may require prolonged or ongoing hospitalisation. This combination of an increasing number of invasive procedures and an ageing, sicker, patient population has meant an associated increase in the incidence of hospital-acquired infections, which significantly increase patient suffering and risk of death, as well as healthcare costs. The most serious form of nosocomial infection is catheter-related bloodstream infection, which involves an infection of the bloodstream secondary to the use of an intravascular catheter.

Nurses are the primary carers of intravascular catheters, and use many strategies in an attempt to prevent catheter-related bloodstream infection (CRBSI). Increasingly, these nursing interventions are being subjected to rigorous testing in an attempt to differentiate EBP from historically based practice. Since 1970, nurses have routinely discarded the administration sets attached to intravenous catheters at regular time intervals, and then replaced them with new sets, in the belief that this may reduce the infection risk. Although several studies showed that infection levels did not differ when the administration sets were replaced at different time intervals, no study had ever been undertaken that measured the value of the practice itself. A recent randomised controlled trial assigned patients to either have their catheter administration sets replaced routinely or to have them left intact, and found no statistically significant difference in infection indicators. The study population comprised high-risk intensive-care patients with short-term (7–10 days) central venous catheters. The results of this study provided Level 1A evidence that the expensive and time-consuming procedure of routine administration set replacement is not effective (Rickard et al in press).

1.9.2 Health-related behaviour evidence

Chronic disease is reaching near-epidemic proportions in the developed world. For example, type 2 diabetes is the fastest growing chronic disease of all, and is rapidly becoming a major health issue for ageing populations due to complications such as blindness, loss of limbs and kidney failure. Most complications are preventable if diabetes is self-managed effectively. However, adequate self-management can be difficult to achieve and maintain for many people because of long-established patterns of health behaviour.

To be effective in improving self-management, nurses working with patients with type 2 diabetes need to understand the role that diabetes plays in people's lives, and why it is that some people continue to not follow their planned diet and undertake regular blood glucose checks, even though they are aware of the possible risks of complications.

1.9.3 Models of nursing care delivery evidence

Since nursing comprises the largest proportion of personnel in the provision of healthcare services, satisfaction with nursing care has been found to be the most important predictor of overall satisfaction with hospital care (Abramowtz et al 1987). Research into the determinants of patient satisfaction with nursing care has been conducted from a variety of perspectives, such as outcome of care and nursing care delivery models (Courtney & Wu 2000). There is a wide evidence base within the management sciences on which nurses may draw to explore issues of quality and organisational design.

1.9.4 Management practice evidence

Historic changes are occurring in the healthcare industry. Programs of managed care, expanding outpatient services and day surgery, cost containment, and demands for efficiency and quality outcomes, are transforming the roles of healthcare providers. These changes have meant nursing executives have had to acquire new skills and competencies to develop a corporate focus. Again, nurses are drawn to the wide management science evidence base in order that they may prepare themselves for the changing roles within their organisations.

1.9.5 Cross-cultural evidence

Nursing care goes far beyond providing a set of treatment interventions. People's experiences, beliefs, attitudes and customs regarding a certain disease or condition can form a stereotype through which physical and emotional sensations may be perceived and interpreted. For example, there is convincing evidence to suggest menopause is experienced differently by many different ethnic groups (Fu et al 2003). For nurses and other health professionals to provide high-quality care to women undergoing menopause, it is important to look to a range of different evidences. Not only is evidence drawn from medicine, but it is also found in the fields of psychology and sociology, as well as exercise-physiology.

1.10 What is the state of evidence?

EBP is undertaken to support the decisions of nurses and other health professionals to avoid the use of not only ineffective, inappropriate and dangerous treatments, but also treatments that have the potential to be unnecessarily costly. Conversely, it is to identify safe, effective and cost-appropriate care. The three-step process through which EBP may be undertaken is described below and is used as an overarching framework for this text.

1.10.1 Step 1: Finding the evidence—how to search for current best evidence

It is important to understand what current best evidence is available and how to find it. However, in order to find the evidence it is essential to know firstly what types of questions to ask. Chapter 2 provides a framework for how to ask research questions and some suggestions for suitable research designs to use in studies to answer such questions. Chapters 3 and 4 provide details of the different types of quantitative and qualitative designs respectively, and why they are undertaken. Additionally, they provide the key features of each design and how they contribute to providing evidence of best practice.

Armed with the right questions and knowledge of the research designs, a comprehensive literature review is undertaken to identify evidence for best practice, and if it is not there, gaps in evidence. Chapter 5 examines systematic reviews of the literature in detail, providing a discussion on what they are, why and how they are undertaken and how they may be used to provide evidence for best practice. This leads to our second step of appraising the evidence.

1.10.2 Step 2: Appraising the evidence—how to critically appraise the evidence

Having undertaken a comprehensive literature search on the effectiveness of a nursing intervention, and found some evidence to suggest its usefulness, it is important to know how to systematically appraise the validity of the research before incorporating it into practice. Additionally assessing the accuracy of diagnostic tests and screening evidence, as well as the validity of the nursing outcomes, is also essential. Chapters 6, 7 and 8 provide details for each of these areas respectively.

1.10.3 Step 3: Using the evidence—how to implement evidence in practice

There are various means by which evidence may be implemented into practice. However, it is important the correct environment is available to do so. Chapter 9 examines the development of a culture of inquiry to sustain EBP and describes characteristics of effective leadership and the role of the organisation in capacity building for change. Chapters 10 and 11 continue with an exploration of how to undertake an audit and evaluation of clinical practice once a culture of inquiry has been developed, while Chapter 12 provides an overview of the development and use of evidence-based guidelines in practice. Finally, the measurement of nursing outcomes is explored in Chapters 13 and 14 by overviewing validated and reliable instruments to measure symptoms and health-related quality of life as nursing outcomes.

1.11 What are the challenges for nursing education and research?

1.11.1 Challenges for nursing research

Over the last decade, the Australian healthcare system has increasingly come under siege to improve the quality and access of patient care within a context of increasingly limited resources. Greater emphasis is being placed on all health professionals to seek out best practice evidence and apply it in their everyday practice.

As there are large gaps in the amount of robust evidence for much of what nurses do during the course of their daily work, the challenge for nurses is to develop, trial, evaluate and implement well-focused evidence-based nursing interventions and treatments to improve the quality of patient care.

1.11.2 Challenges for nursing education

Academic schools of nursing are charged with the responsibility of ensuring nursing graduates are adequately prepared to deliver best practice. Although undergraduate nursing education has been present within universities in Australia for over 25 years, some may question the extent to which an evidence-based culture is embedded within curricula. Indeed, nursing registration authorities require that current best practice for nursing interventions and treatments be included in curricula and that research methods be undertaken.

However, a major challenge for academics is actually teaching EBP throughout a curricula rather than teaching one stand-alone unit usually titled 'Research methods in nursing', which incorporates some EBP content. In order that students be immersed in an evidence-based culture, content on the manner through which evidence may be found, appraised and used in practice should be incorporated very early in curricula and then interwoven throughout every unit of study in the full three years of the course.

1.12 Discussion questions

1. How do you define evidence-based nursing?
2. Why do nurses need good evidence for clinical practice?
3. Where and how can nurses find quality evidence to inform their practice?
4. Briefly list 10 commonly used nursing interventions/procedures/protocols used during the course of your everyday practice. Describe what types of evidence these are based upon (i.e. research study, textbook, experience or opinion).

1.13 References

Abramowtz S, Cote A A, Berry E 1987 Analysing patient satisfaction: a multi-analytic approach. *Quality Research Bulletin* 13(4):122–30.

Anderson D 1998 *Responses to the menopause: hormone replacement therapy and alternatives.* Department of Social and Preventive Medicine, Queensland.

Baker S R, Stacy M C 1994 Epidemiology of chronic leg ulcers in Australia. *Australian and New Zealand Journal of Surgery* 64(4):258–61.

Berwick D M 1998 Developing and testing changes in the delivery of care. *Annals of Internal Medicine* 128(8):651–6.

Bury T J, Mead J M (eds) 1998 *Evidence-based healthcare: a practical guide for therapists.* Butterworth-Heinemann, Oxford.

Chaloner D, Noirit J 1997 Treatments and healing rates in a community leg ulcer clinic. *British Journal of Nursing* 6(5):246–52.

Cochrane Collection website at www.nicsl.com.au/cochrane. Accessed 20 March 2004.

Courtney M, Min Lin Wu 2000 Models of nursing care: a comparative study of patient satisfaction on two orthopaedic wards in Brisbane. *Australian Journal of Advanced Nursing* 17(4):29–34.

Courtney M, Yacopetti J, James C et al 2002 Comparison of the roles and the professional development needs of nurse executives working in metropolitan, provincial, rural and remote settings in Queensland. *Australian Journal of Rural Health* 10(4):202–8.

Craig J V 2002 *The evidence-based practice manual for nurses.* Churchill Livingstone, London.

Dorman M C, Moffatt C J, Franks P J 1995 A model for change in delivering community leg ulcer care. *Ostomy Wound Management* 41(9):34–6, 38–40, 42.

Edwards H, Courtney M, Wilson J et al 2003 Fever management audit: Australian nurses' antipyretic usage. *Paediatric Nursing* 29(1):31–7.

Franks P J 1994 Community leg ulcer clinics: effect on quality of life. *Phlebology* 9(2):83–6.

Fu S-Y, Anderson D, Courtney M 2003 Cross-cultural menopausal experience: comparison of Australian and Taiwanese women. *Nursing and Health Sciences* 5:77–84.

Giacomini M K, Cook D J 2000a Users' guide to the medical literature, XXII: qualitative research in health care. Are the results of the study valid? Evidence Based Medicine Working Group, *JAMA: Journal of the American Medical Association* 284(3):357–62.

Giacomini M K, Cook D J 2000b Users' guide to the medical literature, XXII: qualitative research in health care. What are the results and how do they help me care for my patients? Evidence Based Medicine Working Group, *JAMA: Journal of the American Medical Association* 284(4):478–82.

Grol R 2001 Successes and failures in the implementation of evidence-based guidelines for clinical practice. *Medical Care* 39(8 Suppl 20):1146–54.

Guyatt G, Rennie D (eds) 2002 *Users' guides to the medical literature: essentials of evidence-based practice.* Evidence Based Medicine Working Group, American Medical Association Press, Chicago.

Hammer S, Collinson G (eds) 1999 *Achieving evidence-based practice: a handbook for practitioners.* Bailliere Tindall, London.

Harrison J E 2000 Evidence-based orthodontics: how do I assess the evidence? *Journal of Orthodontics* 27(2):189–97.

Johnson M 1995 The prevalence of leg ulcers in older people: implications for community nursing. *Public Health Nursing* 12(4):269–75.

Lees T A, Lambert D 1992 Prevalence of lower limb ulceration in an urban health district. *British Journal of Surgery* 79(10):1032–4.

Lindsay E 2000 Leg clubs: A new approach to patient-centred leg ulcer management. *Nursing and Health Sciences* 2:139–41.

Lockett T 1997 Traces of evidence. *Healthcare Today* July/August:16.

National Health Service (NHS) website at www.modern.nhs.uk. Accessed 20 March 2004.

National Health Service (NHS) Centre for Reviews and Dissemination 1999 Getting evidence into practice. *Effective Healthcare* 5(1):1–16.

National Institute of Clinical Studies (NICS) 2003 *Evidence–practice gaps report vol 1.* NICS, Melbourne.

National Institute for Clinical Studies (NICS) 2004 Adopting best evidence in practice. *Medical Journal of Australia* 180(6):s41–2.

National Institute for Clinical Studies (NICS) website at www.nicsl.com.au. Accessed 20 March 2004.

Queensland Health 2003 *Clinician development program education service.* Queensland Health, Brisbane.

Rickard C, Lipman J, Courtney M et al 2004 Routine changing of intravascular administration-sets does not reduce colonization or infection in central venous catheters. *Infection Control and Hospital Epidemiology* (in press accepted February 2004).

Russell G, Bowles A 1992 Developing a community-based leg ulcer clinic. *British Journal of Nursing* 1(7):337–40.

Sackett D L, Straus S E, Richardson W S et al 1997 *Evidence based medicine: how to practice and teach EBM*, 1st edn. Churchill Livingstone, London.

Sackett D L, Straus S E, Richardson W S et al 2000 *Evidence based medicine: how to practice and teach EBM*, 2nd edn. Churchill Livingstone, London.

Schuster M, McGlynn E, Brook R H 1988 How good is the quality of healthcare in the United States? *Millbank Quarterly* 76:517–63.

Silagy C 2001 Evidence-based healthcare 10 years on: is the National Institute of Clinical Studies the answer? (editorial). *Medical Journal of Australia* 175:124–5.

Tarling M, Crofts L 1998 *The essential researcher's handbook for nurses and healthcare professionals*, 1st edn. Bailliere Tindall, London.

Tarling M, Crofts L 2002 *The essential researcher's handbook for nurses and healthcare professionals*, 2nd edn. Bailliere Tindall, London.

Thurlby K, Griffiths P 2002 Community leg ulcer clinics vs home visits: which is more effective? *British Journal of Community Nursing* 7(5):260–5.

appendix (1.1)

National Institute for Clinical Studies: clinical priority areas

In many areas of healthcare there are clear gaps between what best research evidence tells us should be done, and what is actually done in everyday clinical care. Studies have shown that between 30% and 40% of patients do not receive care based on best research evidence, and 20–30% of the care provided is not needed or is potentially harmful (Schuster et al 1988, Grol 2001).

The National Institute of Clinical Studies (NICS) was established in 2001 as Australia's national agency for improving healthcare by helping close these important gaps. One of its primary goals is to increase knowledge about the science and art of evidence uptake in clinical care.

Evidence—practice gaps

One of the first tasks undertaken by the NICS was to identify important evidence–practice gaps in Australia. In its first year of operation NICS conducted an extensive consultation process, seeking the views of medical, nursing and allied health clinicians throughout Australia. This consultation process (the gaps analysis), supported by a variety of literature reviews, led to the identification of a number of clinical areas where there were demonstrable gaps between research and practice.

Later work undertaken by the NICS attempted a different approach, linking identified best practice to actual practice data. What soon became clear was that while there is ample evidence to support what should be done in practice it is often difficult to find data to show what actually takes place in everyday practice. This means that we do not always know whether patients are getting the care that will deliver the best outcomes for them.

Despite these limitations the NICS was able to identify a number of evidence–practice gaps in the first of a projected series of publications, which describe these gaps in the Australian context (NICS 2003). They include things that are done for which there is no sound evidence, such as screening for lung cancer with chest X-rays, bowel cleansing prior to colorectal surgery, and prescribing antibiotics for the common cold and acute bronchitis. The gaps also include things that should be done but which are not done enough, such as measuring glycated haemoglobin in diabetes management, intervening to prevent thromboembolism in hospitalised patients, and prescribing anticoagulants to help prevent stroke in patients with atrial fibrillation. The gaps also include things that are generally done poorly, such as managing acute and cancer pain in hospitalised patients and providing advice on smoking cessation in both general practice and antenatal care.

Methods

In undertaking the challenge of clinical practice change the NICS has adopted a number of methods to engage both clinicians and Australian healthcare users.

Improving implementation of clinical practice guidelines

Clinical practice guidelines have been a mainstay of attempts to get evidence into clinical practice. Notwithstanding the many problems with the guideline production process (such as source reliability, currency and local applicability), there are still significant barriers to their use in everyday practice.

The NICS is a founding member of the Guidelines International Network (G-I-N—see www.g-i-n.net), a 50-member international network that seeks to 'improve the quality of healthcare by promoting systematic development of clinical practice guidelines and their application into practice through supporting international collaboration'. The NICS will be working within G-I-N to identify more effective ways to incorporate evidence-based clinical guidelines in healthcare.

Identification of leaders

Fostering clinical leadership is a strategy adopted by the NICS as a way of encouraging clinically relevant and applicable evidence uptake. The NICS fellowship program was launched in 2003 and aims to identify future clinical leaders from a variety of backgrounds and disciplines, who are then mentored and supported to undertake clinical improvement projects. Current fellows are undertaking work on strategies for increasing use of the most appropriate venous access for renal dialysis, on ways to increase prescription of warfarin to patients with atrial fibrillation and supporting EBP in rural emergency departments. The NICS has also assisted clinical leadership in the primary care sector through General Practice Leaders awards, which provide opportunities for general practitioners and practice nurses to receive training to implement clinical improvement projects in primary care.

Publication and promotion of synthesised work

To support Australian clinicians to increase the use of EBP the NICS has commissioned a number of literature reviews that examine successful strategies that have been used to achieve this aim. The scope of the reviews is diverse and reflects the wide range of information the NICS has incorporated into its programs. Three reviews illustrate this range. In 'Factors supporting high performance in health care organisation' the reviewers identify the prerequisites (goal setting and feedback, leadership and human resources management), enablers (structure, climate and culture) and drivers (organisational learning and knowledge transfer, training and development, and quality management) that are present in healthcare organisations that perform well. In 'Institutional approaches to pain assessment and management' the reviewers attempt to identify whether embedding pain assessment in the organisational structure of a health service is successful and sustainable. The review 'Thromboembolism prophylaxis in hospitals' critically evaluates strategies used to increase uptake of prophylaxis in at-risk patients. These and other reviews are available at www.nicsl.com.au.

Web and literature searching

As a service to the Australian clinical community the NICS regularly monitors a number of current journals and websites to identify strategies that have been tried to increase uptake of evidence, or to highlight areas of interest. Reports are periodically posted on the NICS website.

Building networks

The NICS has forged close links and working relationships with a number of Australia's peak health bodies, colleges, professional associations and researchers, and with international academics and researchers.

In 2003 the NICS invited many of Australia's healthcare, social science, clinical and consumer opinion leaders to a workshop in Hobart to discuss approaches to improving evidence uptake across the Australian healthcare system. The workshop identified a number of primary care, community and hospital approaches that the NICS is further investigating and considering (NICS 2004a).

The NICS is investigating the effectiveness of clinical networks and communities of practice as two promising vehicles for evidence-based clinical change. Communities of practice, defined as networks established to increase and promote the sharing and use of information and problem solving in groups with a common interest, have been used extensively in the information technology and engineering professions, and a NICS project using this approach in the emergency care sector is underway.

Tools

The NICS has worked closely with other organisations to assist Australian healthcare professionals to access evidence for clinical decision making.

The Cochrane Library

Clinician access to high-quality, appraised clinical evidence is a prerequisite for EBP. The Cochrane Library is recognised as one of the best sources of such evidence on clinical interventions. In 2001 an open access agreement to the Cochrane Library was negotiated by the NICS on behalf of the Australian Government for all Australian residents. Recognising that, because of its origins as an academic research tool, the Cochrane Library interface presents problems for many would-be users, the NICS worked with the Australasian Cochrane Centre to produce a comprehensive web-based users' guide to the Library (see www.nicsl.com.au/cochrane).

In another initiative to promote usage of the Library the NICS offers annual awards to Australian clinicians who have accessed the Library and have been able to demonstrate subsequent benefits for patients. The winning entries for 2003 included a midwifery team that designed evidence-based perinatal care guidelines and trialled methods for integrating the guidelines into everyday practice in 20 midwifery units. Further initiatives reduced the incidence of post-partum haemorrhage and reduced the incidence of deep-vein thrombosis and pulmonary embolism in a hospital. A prize was also awarded to the developers of a program to increase mobility and presurgery fitness for patients prior to joint replacement surgery. All the winners had designed and instituted clinical interventions based on the findings of Cochrane Library reviews.

Electronic decision support

Electronic decision support (EDS), defined as 'a system that compares patient characteristics with a knowledge base and then guides a health provider by offering patient specific and situation specific advice' (Friedman & Wyatt 1977), is a common medium for disseminating evidence into practice. While there are a number of EDS products available to Australian clinicians, there has been concern from many quarters that these tools are being developed and offered without an overarching governance structure in place to ensure quality and adherence to evidence-based principles.

In a workshop in 2001 the NICS, in conjunction with the National Health Information Management Advisory Council, drew together a number of key players from industry, government and clinical practice to debate the problem (NICS 2002). As a result of the workshop the Australian Government established an Electronic Decision Support Task Force to recommend the way ahead for ensuring a national approach to the development of EDS systems (Electronic Decision Support Task Force 2002). The NICS is currently funding a major research project that seeks to identify current use of EDS and barriers to EDS use in clinical practice, in response to one of the Task Force's key recommendations.

Four evidence–practice gaps

As a result of its gaps consultation process the NICS identified four key clinical areas for engagement. In each there is a demonstrable gap between evidence and practice, and an opportunity for the NICS to examine one or a combination of change strategies.

Area 1: improving chronic heart failure management

Chronic heart failure is a significant clinical problem in Australia, affecting an estimated 325,000 people, with a further 200,000 people estimated to have heart failure without overt symptoms (Stewart et al 2003). As in many developed countries, the incidence is expected to rise given an ageing population.

The fundamental principle of the NICS heart failure strategy is the acknowledgment that a chronic disease like heart failure is an entire health system condition, managed at the general practice, community and hospital level, as well as involving decision makers at government level. The approach taken by the NICS was to identify the most important gaps at each level of influence on heart failure management in Australia, from government to clinician to individual patient. The NICS is advised by a number of cardiologists, general practitioners, nurses, pharmacists and consumer representatives in the field of heart failure, and works closely with the National Heart Foundation of Australia and the National Prescribing Service (Australia's national agency for providing independent pharmaceutical information).

Three important issues have been identified. The first of these relates to diagnosis. Clinical diagnosis of chronic heart failure is often unreliable, especially in obese patients, those with lung disease and the elderly. The current recommended investigation for the diagnosis of suspected heart failure is echocardiography, yet many patients are still diagnosed without the objective measurement of ventricular function that echocardiography can offer.

The second issue relates to treatment. There is evidence from Australia and overseas that many patients are treated suboptimally with two classes of medications considered the current gold standard of heart failure therapy (Krum 2001), angiotensin-converting enzyme (ACE) inhibitors and beta blockers, and that some patients are not prescribed them at all (Krum et al 2001, Scott et al 2003). In Australia the barriers to prescription exist at both a health system level (e.g. for some time general practitioners had been unable to prescribe certain types of drugs, as government had restricted their use in the national drug formulary), and at individual prescriber level.

The third issue relates to patient self-management. There is ample evidence to suggest that interventions such as daily weighing and telephone contact with specialist cardiac nurses can prevent exacerbation of symptoms, which in turn can prevent unnecessary presentations to hospital emergency departments. Despite this, many patients are unaware of the role they can play in the management of their own condition.

The heart failure program will trial three forms of intervention. In the area of diagnostics the NICS has undertaken research that has identified barriers to the uptake of echocardiography from the general practice sector (Phillips et al in press) (which include difficulty accessing services, particularly in rural Australia, and uncertainty about the value of echocardiography itself), and will work with other professional groups to trial the use of education modules and small interactive sessions with general practitioners to increase echocardiography uptake. In the area of treatment the National Prescribing Service will use the technique of academic detailing in general practices that service populations with high proportions of elderly people.

In the area of self-management the program addresses the paucity of high-quality, evidence-based consumer-focused information for heart failure patients. Research commissioned by the NICS reviewed Australian materials on heart failure and surveyed health professionals and consumer groups' needs. A number of resources were identified and assessed using the 'checklist for assessing written consumer health information' (Currie et al 2000). The study found that most clinicians and consumer groups wanted more help in locating and accessing quality resources. The NICS developed an online directory of the highest quality evidence-based resources identified in response to the needs of participants, and this can be accessed at www.nicsl.com.au.

Area 2: emergency department care

Hospital emergency departments can often act as a barometer of the health of a system and the problems of access block, ambulance bypass and inappropriate presentation have been an important issue in most Australian states and territories for a number of years.

Consultations revealed a number of evidence–practice gaps in Australian hospital emergency care, and the NICS worked closely with a number of state governments and nursing and medical organisations to address these gaps in the first national initiative of its kind in Australia.

The NICS consultations confirmed that international research reflected problems in Australian emergency departments. A key gap identified was the length of time patients had to wait before being given pain relief. American research has shown that as many as 78% of patients presenting to emergency departments have pain as their main complaint (Tanabe & Buschmann 1999). While Australian guidelines suggest that early pain management is usually warranted in emergency care (NHMRC 1999) a literature review commissioned by the NICS identified Israeli research showing that time to analgesia can range from 30 to 140 minutes from arrival in emergency departments (Zohar et al 2002). Delays in administering analgesia are commonly attributed to factors such as fear of compromising diagnosis, unavailability of nurses to cannulate and lack of space to observe patients after they have been given pain relief.

Other evidence–practice gaps identified included delays in administering thrombolysis to patients presenting with myocardial infarction (where evidence shows that the optimal treatment time is within one hour of first symptoms), delays in administration of antibiotics for patients with febrile neutropenia and community-acquired pneumonia, and problems with patient flow through emergency departments.

In undertaking work to bridge the gaps the NICS tested the 'plan–do–study–act' or 'breakthrough collaborative' clinical improvement model. This model has been used extensively in healthcare throughout the world, in settings ranging from individual health facilities to, in the case of the English National Health Service Modernisation Agency, an entire country. The model is based on serial small-scale incremental improvements and was promoted and has been vigorously championed by Don Berwick of the American Institute of Healthcare Improvement (Berwick 1998). At the time of writing about 20 large-scale collaboratives had been run in Australia alone since 2001.

The NICS project was the first national collaborative and involved 47 hospitals from most states and territories in Australia. All tackled time to analgesia as a key indicator and each chose a number of others relevant to local priorities.

Although the collaborative model is widely used, there is still much to be learnt about the longer term effectiveness of the model, particularly in relation to sustainability of change. The NICS commissioned a number of evaluation research studies to run parallel with the collaborative. One project measured the relationship between the 'culture' within an emergency department and its ability to achieve change, using proprietary Change-Tracking® methodology. Another will revisit the emergency departments one year after the collaborative to measure the sustainability of change.

The collaborative ran from May 2003 until October 2003. There were substantial improvements in measured time to pain relief in a third of the participating hospitals and a patient satisfaction survey showed that patients noticed improvements in their care and their pain management. Staff job satisfaction and workplace culture improved during the collaborative (NICS 2004a). It was observed that since the end of the collaborative some hospitals have adapted the breakthrough methodology to tackle other problems in their departments.

While the usefulness of the breakthrough collaborative as a long-term quality improvement strategy is still under evaluation, the NICS is continuing to work in the field of emergency care, broadening the boundaries beyond the emergency department itself. In order to do this, the NICS will trial the communities of practice model. The four key objectives of the community will be to assist the uptake of EBP in emergency care, to identify common challenges, to provide access to good quality evidence-based materials and solutions, and to develop processes for making best use of good quality clinical care data.

Area 3: improving pain management

The nursing reference group established by the NICS was asked to identify clinical priority areas of relevance to nursing where strong evidence–practice gaps exist in Australia. The group identified the assessment and treatment of pain as problematic in a number of institutional settings in Australia, including paediatrics, residential aged care (McLean & Higginbotham 2002) and cancer treatment (Yates et al 2002).

Current information suggests that unrelieved cancer pain is a significant problem. The International Association for the Study of Pain collected data on pain in 1095 cancer patients across 24 countries, including Australia. All patients were already prescribed opioid analgesia, yet 53% rated their average pain as moderate to severe and 65% were experiencing breakthrough pain (Caraceni & Portenoy 1999). Australian studies indicate that pain in hospitalised cancer patients is prevalent. One study of 93 cancer patients in an Australian teaching hospital found that one-third had moderate to severe pain (Potter et al 2003), while another study of 114 cancer patients in two Australian hospitals found that 48% reported pain and 44% of these had moderate to severe pain (Yates et al 2002).

Best available evidence suggests that cancer pain can be well controlled in 80–90% of patients when treatment is tailored to individual circumstances (Zech et al 1995), yet the established attitudes, practices and beliefs of both healthcare professionals and patients often hinder effective pain relief, and many patients suffer unnecessarily. Healthcare professionals outside of specialist pain services do not routinely assess or document pain (Manias 2003), frequently underestimate patients' pain levels (Chan & Woodruff 1997) and are inconsistent and conservative in their approach to analgesic medications.

Organisation-wide quality improvement programs to implement generic pain management standards have been advocated to reduce barriers, improve practice and lessen the burden of pain in hospitals. In 2004 the NICS launched a pilot pain-management program to test system-wide intervention. The objective of the program is to establish an institutional commitment to effective routine pain management at the organisational, clinical and consumer levels in a small number of major hospitals. The specific aims relate to improving the day-to-day assessment and management of pain, focusing on cancer services and units.

Area 4: venous thromboembolism prevention

The incidence of venous thromboembolism in hospitalised patients is around 135 times greater compared to the general community (Heit et al 2002), and there are approximately 16,000 hospitalisations in Australia each year where deep-vein thrombosis is reported and 14,000 where pulmonary embolism is reported. The latter is one of the single most common preventable causes of death in hospital, accounting for or contributing to 10% of all deaths in hospital.

Preventing deep-vein thrombosis in high-risk patients (those undergoing orthopaedic and neurosurgery, and many patients with cancer) is based on heparin and compression stockings. The NICS has drawn together a number of hospital audits and published studies on venous thromboembolism prevention in Australia and, while the picture varies significantly between hospitals and types of patient, one small study showed the prophylaxis rate for high-risk patients in one hospital to be only 5%. A previous national audit of surgical care in the early 1990s showed the prophylaxis rates for patients undergoing hip and knee surgery in Australia and New Zealand were 65% and 39% respectively (Fletcher et al 2002).

As previously stated, one of the problems with defining evidence–practice gaps in Australia is the lack of routine clinical data available to monitor practice. Thromboembolism prophylaxis is a good illustration of this problem. Because deep-vein thrombosis and pulmonary embolism are commonly secondary complications of an existing hospital admission rather than the main cause of hospitalisation, data collected in Australia under the International Classification of Disease system (where only the principal diagnosis is collected) may miss these incidents, and treatment data may become more difficult to find. Another problem is that as deep-vein thrombosis may occur several months after hospital discharge, the link between an original condition and the later complication may not be made. Further complicating matters, routinely collected data on low-molecular-weight heparin prescribing in Australia does not specifically distinguish between prophylactic and therapeutic usage.

In this project the NICS is investigating the use of data linkage (formally linking otherwise unconnected data sources) to try to overcome some of the problems lack of clinical practice data presents. This has the potential to provide a unique picture of the risk of developing deep-vein thrombosis and pulmonary embolism following hospital admission, and to provide better data on the long-term effectiveness of thromboembolism prophylaxis strategies post-hospital discharge. This will assist the NICS to better target interventions for at-risk patients.

The science of evidence-based implementation of evidence-based care

Underpinning all the initiatives the NICS has undertaken to date is an emphasis on increasing our understanding of the evidence base of changing clinical behaviour, identifying what works and what does not work in a scientific manner. This is a new and emerging field for, as Grimshaw and Eccles (2004) have noted, there is a 'lack of a robust theoretical base for understanding healthcare provider and organisational behaviour'.

The NICS has taken a number of approaches to doing this, including look-ing to industries other than health (such as mining and aviation) where improvements in safety have been achieved through firmly embedding change culture into organisational structures. Experts in the psychology of behavioural change advise the NICS on all aspects of its work program and all clinical intervention programs have rigorous built-in evaluation strategies.

In the longer term it is the intention of the NICS to publish widely on what works to change clinician and organisational behaviour in the Australian setting. In the interim the NICS has commissioned a number of local and overseas experts to summarise the overseas experience of getting evidence into practice (NICS 2004b), and continues to invite overseas experts in health system change to Australia.

Conclusion

During its relatively short existence the NICS has done much to identify and address some of the major gaps between evidence and best practice in Australia. By working closely with the doctors, nurses, allied health profes-sionals, policy makers and consumers who make up the healthcare sector in Australia, the NICS is uniquely placed, through its growing expertise in the science of change management, to help bridge many of the gaps that have been identified so far.

References

Berwick D M 1998 Developing and testing changes in the delivery of care. *Annals of Internal Medicine* 128(8):651–6.

Caraceni A, Portenoy R K 1999 An international survey of cancer pain characteristics and syndromes. IASP task force on cancer pain. International Association for the Study of Pain. *Pain* 82:263–74.

Chan A, Woodruff R K 1997 Communicating with patients with advanced cancer. *Journal of Palliative Care* 13:29–33.

Currie K, Spink J, Rajendran M 2000 *Communicating with consumers series volume one. Well-written health information: a guide.* July, Department of Human Services, Melbourne.

Fletcher J P, Koutts J, Ockelford P A 2002 Deep vein thrombosis prophylaxis: a survey of current practice in Australia and New Zealand. *Australia & New Zealand Journal of Surgery* 62:601–5.

Friedman C P, Wyatt J C 1977 *Evaluation methods in medical infomatics.* Springer-Verlag, New York.

Grimshaw J M, Eccles M P 2004 Is evidence-based implementation of evidence-based care possible? *Medical Journal of Australia* 180:s50–1.

Grol R 2001 Successes and failures in the implementation of evidence-based guidelines for clinical practice. *Medical Care* 39(8 Suppl 20):1146–54.

Heit J A, Melton L J 3rd, Lohse C M et al 2002 Incidence of venous thromboembolism in hospitalised patients vs community residents. *Mayo Clinic Proceedings* 76:1102–10.

Krum H 2001 National Heart Foundation of Australia and Cardiac Society of Australia & New Zealand Chronic Heart Failure Clinical Practice Guidelines Writing Panel. Guidelines for management of patients with chronic heart failure in Australia. *Medical Journal of Australia* 174:459–66.

Krum H, Tonkin A M, Currie R et al 2001 Chronic heart failure in Australian general practice. The cardiac awareness survey and evaluation (CASE) study. *Medical Journal of Australia* 174:439–44.

Manias E 2003 Medication trends and documentation of pain management following surgery. *Nursing & Health Sciences* 5:85–94.

McLean W J, Higginbotham N H 2002 Prevalence of pain among nursing home residents in rural New South Wales. *Australian Medical Journal* 177:17–20.

National Electronic Decision Support Taskforce 2002 *Electronic decision support for Australia's health sector.* Commonwealth of Australia, Canberra.

National Health and Medical Research Institute (NHMRC) 1999 *Acute pain management: scientific evidence.* NHMRC Report, Commonwealth of Australia, Canberra.

National Institute of Clinical Studies (NICS) 2002 *Report of the electronic decision support governance workshop.* NICS, Melbourne. Available at www.nicsl.com.au.

National Institute of Clinical Studies (NICS) 2003 *Evidence–practice gaps report volume 1.* NICS, Melbourne.

National Institute of Clinical Studies (NICS) 2004a Adopting best evidence in practice. *Medical Journal of Australia* 180(6):s41–72.

National Institute of Clinical Studies (NICS) 2004b *National emergency department collaborative report October 2002–October 2003.* NICS, Melbourne. Available at www.nicsl.com.au.

Phillips S M, Marton R L, Tofler G H Barriers to the diagnosis and management of heart failure in primary care. *Medical Journal of Australia* (in press).

Potter V T, Wiseman C E, Dunn S M, Boyle F M 2003 Patient barriers to optimal cancer pain control. *Psycho-Oncology* 12:153–60.

Schuster M, McGlynn E, Brook R H 1988 How good is the quality of health care in the United States? *Millbank Quarterly* 76:517–63.

Scott I A, Denaro C P, Flores J L et al 2003 Quality of care of patients hospitalised with congestive heart failure. *Internal Medicine Journal* 33:140–51.

Stewart S, McLennon S, Dawson A, Clarke R 2003 *Uncovering a hidden epidemic: a study of the current burden of heart failure in Australia.* Centre for Innovation in Health, University of South Australia, Adelaide. Available at www.unisa.edu.au/hsc/events.htm.

Tanabe P, Buschmann M 1999 A prospective study of ED pain management practices and the patient's perspective. *Journal of Emergency Nursing* 25(3):171–7.

Yates P M, Edwards H E, Nash R E et al 2002 Barriers to effective pain management: a survey of hospitalised cancer patients in Australia. *Journal of Pain & Symptom Management* 23:393–405.

Zech D F, Grond S, Lynch J et al 1995 Validation of World Health Organization guidelines for cancer pain relief: a 10 year prospective study. *Pain* 63:65–76.

Zohar et al 2002, cited in *Early pain management in the hospital emergency department: a critical literature review.* Available at www.nicsl.com.au.

Joanna Briggs Institute Collaborating Centres

In addition to the JBI Collaborating Centres listed below, new Centres are also planned in Sweden, the United States of America, China (Shanghai), India, Japan and Italy.

Australia

The Queensland Centre for Evidence Based Nursing and Midwifery: A Collaborating Centre of the Joanna Briggs Institute, Mater Hospital, Brisbane

The Australian Centre for Evidence Based Rural Health: A Collaborating Centre of the Joanna Briggs Institute, University of Southern Queensland, Toowoomba

The Australian Centre for Evidence Based Nutrition and Dietetics: A Collaborating Centre of the Joanna Briggs Institute, University of Newcastle, Newcastle

The New South Wales Centre for Evidence Based Healthcare: A Collaborating Centre of the Joanna Briggs Institute, University of Western Sydney, Sydney

The Australian Centre for Evidence Based Aged Care: A Collaborating Centre of the Joanna Briggs Institute, La Trobe University, Melbourne

The Victorian Centre for Evidence Based Nursing and Midwifery: A Collaborating Centre of the Joanna Briggs Institute, University of Melbourne, Melbourne

The Centre for Allied Health Evidence: A Collaborating Centre of the Joanna Briggs Institute, University of South Australia, Adelaide

The Centre for Evidence Based Nursing South Australia: A Collaborating Centre of the Joanna Briggs Institute, University of Adelaide, Adelaide

The Western Australian Centre for Evidence Based Nursing and Midwifery: A Collaborating Centre of the Joanna Briggs Institute, Curtin University, Perth

Canada

The Centre for Evidence Based Nursing: A Collaborating Centre of the Joanna Briggs Institute, Queens University, Kingston, Ontario

New Zealand

Centre for Evidence Based Nursing Aotearoa (CEBNA): A Collaborating Centre of the Joanna Briggs Institute, University of Auckland, Auckland

Europe

The Centre for Evidence Based Nursing: A Collaborating Centre of the Joanna Briggs Institute, University of Nottingham, England

The Centre for Evidence Based Healthcare: A Collaborating Centre of the Joanna Briggs Institute, Robert Gordon University, Aberdeen, Scotland

The Centre for Evidence Based Midwifery: A Collaborating Centre of the Joanna Briggs Institute, Thames Valley University, England

The Spanish Centre for Evidence Based Nursing and Midwifery: A Collaborating Centre of the Joanna Briggs Institute, Madrid, Spain

South Africa

The South African Centre for Evidence Based Nursing: A Collaborating Centre of the Joanna Briggs Institute, University of Natal, Durban

South-East Asia

The Hong Kong Centre for Evidence Based Nursing: A Collaborating Centre of the Joanna Briggs Institute, Chinese University of Hong Kong, Hong Kong, SAR, Peoples Republic of China

The Thailand Centre for Evidence Based Nursing and Midwifery: A Collaborating Centre of the Joanna Briggs Institute, Chiang Mai University, Chiang Mai, Thailand

part two ◎—●

How to search for current best evidence

chapter ② ──────────●

Using the right type of evidence to answer clinical questions

Joan Webster and Sonya Osborne

2.1 Learning objectives

After reading this chapter, you should be able to:

1. *categorise a clinical question in terms of whether it relates to intervention/therapy, frequency, diagnosis, prognosis/harm or to understanding phenomena*
2. *describe the most appropriate type of study required to answer a clinical question, and*
3. *understand the use of hierarchies of evidence for studies that measure the effect of an intervention.*

2.2 Introduction

The 1997–98 Federal Government Budget announced a measure aimed at improving health outcomes for patients by ensuring that new and existing medical procedures are supported by scientific evidence (Australian Government 1997). In support of the measure, funding was provided for the establishment of a new body, the Medical Services Advisory Committee. The role of the Committee was to assemble and review available evidence to establish the safety, clinical effectiveness and cost effectiveness of medical interventions. Although the use of evidence-based practice (EBP) to improve disease treatment and prevention is not new, the Federal Government's initiative placed EBP firmly on the agenda of state health departments and this has been reflected in their strategic directions and health plans (NSW Health 2000, Queensland Health 2003b). It also provided the policy context for EBP, including evidence-based nursing in Australia.

Despite this, wide-scale use of research evidence to underpin nursing practice has been difficult to achieve (Foxcroft 2003), and even the most basic interventions, such as pressure area care, still lack an evidence base (Gould et al 2000). Reasons for this are discussed in other chapters, but one limitation is an understanding (or lack of understanding) about what constitutes 'scientific evidence' and confusion about the types of evidence that are required to answer particular research questions. The purpose of this chapter is to focus on evidence and its meaning in the context of nursing practice.

2.3 Types of evidence

The notion that most nursing practice is experimental may come as a surprise to many nurses. There is a general belief that 'evidence' exists for nursing interventions and that what we do in our day-to-day work is beneficial for patients. In reality, if one considers evidence to be the use of research that is based on rigorous epidemiological methods and has been published in peer-reviewed journals, there is no evidence of effect, either harm or benefit, for most nursing procedures. This is largely because nurses have been reluctant or unable to employ the type of research methods where groups of patients are systematically exposed to alternative interventions, so that the effectiveness of various approaches may be evaluated. Rather, nurses have tended to use past experience, peer opinion or policies to inform their day-to-day practice (Hicks 1998). This approach becomes difficult when the view of one 'expert' differs from another, or where policies and guidelines are not based on well-appraised or systematically reviewed evidence.

It is a hackneyed expression to say that 'the type of research design depends on the type of question asked', but it is amazing how many examples can be found in the literature where the wrong study type has been used when attempting to answer a particular question. The fallout from this is that when seeking strong evidence to support a particular nursing practice, we constantly run into brick walls. In this chapter, we will focus on the types of questions nurses may ask to inform their practice and the types of research evidence required to answer those questions (Table 2.1 summarises this information).

Table 2.1 Finding the best evidence by using the correct study type

Type of question	Explanation	Type of study (i.e. type of evidence)
Intervention/therapy	How can we alleviate the problem?	• Systematic review of all randomised controlled trials • Randomised controlled trial • Cohort study • Case controlled study
Frequency	What is the prevalence of the problem?	• Cross-sectional survey (prevalence study) or census
Diagnosis (test accuracy) (screening)	Does this person have the problem?	• Systematic review • Random sample or consecutive sample compared with a 'gold standard' test • Randomised controlled trial
Prognosis/aetiology/harm	Who will get the problem, or what caused the problem?	• Follow-up of inception cohort • Case-controlled study
Phenomena	What are the phenomena or problems?	• Observational/qualitative

Source: Adapted from Queensland Health 2003a.

2.3.1 Intervention/treatment/therapy questions (questions about effect)

A recent survey of doctors who contacted a telephone service that was designed to find rapid answers to their queries showed that questions about intervention/treatment or therapy were the most common (Brassey et al 2001). Although there is no comparable published data for nurses, results would probably be similar. One could imagine, in a climate where there is less and less time to provide patient care, that it would be useful to know which of the interventions or therapies employed by nurses every day in their practice are effective and which are not. We need this information to be able to efficiently prioritise time and to make the best use of available resources. One way to determine whether or not a question falls into this category is to ask: 'Does this nursing care practice help alleviate the patient's problem or prevent a problem from occurring?' For example:

- Does wearing a gown prevent nosocomial infection in neonatal nurseries?
- Do smoking cessation programs delivered by nurses lead to lower tobacco use?
- Do pressure reduction mattresses reduce the incidence of pressure ulcers?
- Do routine observations lead to earlier diagnosis of complications?

A number of study types (types of evidence) may be used to answer intervention or therapy questions but the randomised controlled trial is considered to be the 'gold standard' of research designs for providing evidence of effect. The randomised controlled trial design is powerful because the randomisation process ensures an unbiased distribution of potential confounders. That is, patients in the intervention group and the control group are equal in all respects except for the intervention being trialled.

Comparing the number of 'events' or 'outcomes' (e.g. number of infections, number of pressure ulcers) in the two groups assesses the relative effectiveness of the intervention. This evidence becomes even more powerful when the results of a number of randomised trials, which have addressed the same question, are combined in a systematic review and/or meta-analysis. For example, if we wanted to know whether silver sulphadiazine was more effective than other topical agents or dressings in limiting infection and facilitating healing in partial and full thickness burns, we would begin by searching for a systematic review of all randomised controlled trials that had addressed this question. If we were able to find such a review (such as a Cochrane Review), and it met quality standards (see an excellent description by Tricia Greenhalgh in the *British Medical Journal* (Greenhalgh 1997b)) we could be reasonably certain that we had found the best source of evidence to answer our question.

If no systematic review were available, we would search for individual randomised controlled trials and assess the quality of the trials using some type of checklist, such as the CONSORT Statement (Begg et al 1996) and its recent revisions (Moher et al 2003) to ensure that the trial was free from major biases. If neither of these types of studies were available, we may consider the results of other studies, those with less strength to answer the research question convincingly.

Several organisations have developed hierarchies of evidence that grade study designs from strongest to weakest—those at the head of the hierarchy are those that are least open to bias. For example, the National Health and Medical Research Council's (NHMRC) table (see Table 2.2) is widely used for this purpose. Other organisations, such as the Oxford Centre for Evidence-based

Medicine, have produced more complex tables of studies that provide levels of evidence for other types of research questions such as those about diagnosis, prognosis, economic and decision analysis, frequency as well as for therapy and intervention questions (see www.cebm.net/levels_of_evidence.asp). There is no doubt that, as the science of EBP continues to develop, such hierarchies of evidence will continue to evolve.

Table 2.2 Grading of research studies that measure the effect of an intervention, treatment or therapy

Level of evidence	Study designs
I	Evidence obtained from a systematic review or meta-analysis of all relevant randomised controlled trials
II	Evidence obtained from at least one properly designed randomised controlled trial
III–1	Evidence obtained from well-designed pseudo-randomised controlled trials (alternate allocation or some other method)
III–2	Evidence obtained from comparative studies with concurrent controls and allocation not randomised (cohort studies, case-control studies or interrupted time-series with control group)
III–3	Evidence obtained from comparative studies with historical control, two or more single-arm studies, or interrupted time-series without a parallel control group
IV	Evidence obtained from case series (either post-test or pretest and post-test)

Source: NHMRC 1999.

The reason why qualitative methods are not included in such hierarchies of evidence has been questioned. For example, Pravikoff and Donaldson (2001) argue that many patient care issues of interest to nurses are not researchable using the randomised controlled trial. We would agree. Qualitative methods are extremely valuable, but they do not measure the effect of an intervention, which all of the studies included in such tables are designed to do. As we will see, they provide evidence to answer different types of research questions, and so do not belong on lists grading a study's efficacy.

There is no good argument for avoiding the use of well-designed controlled clinical trials to test the validity of nursing interventions or nursing practices whenever possible. They are the principal means of ensuring that such interventions are useful, cost effective and safe. For example, Moore and colleagues have shown that outcomes for patients visiting either a nurse continence adviser or a urogynaecologist for conservative management of urinary incontinence were equivalent, but treatment costs were substantially less when provided by the nurse (Moore et al 2003). Similarly, nurse-led telephone consultations with people with asthma compared with face-to-face consultations in the surgery enabled more people with asthma to be reviewed, without clinical disadvantage or loss of satisfaction (Pinnock et al 2003).

In a further example, nurses were shown to be as effective as house officers in assessing patients, in terms of history taking and physical assessment, before general anaesthesia for surgery (Kinley et al 2002). In this study, nurses also ordered less unnecessary tests than house officers. As we move into an era of nurse practitioners, having information from such trials and using randomised controlled trial methodology to test the effectiveness of nursing interventions in other areas of practice is essential. Conversely the randomised controlled trial is extremely important for identifying practices that are time-consuming or costly yet have no evidence of effect. For example, the benefit of a nurse-led program to assist pregnant women to quit smoking and prevent relapse was found to be ineffective when compared with the normal care approach (Moore et al 2002). The authors acknowledged that providing accurate information about the effects of smoking in pregnancy was important; however, they showed that spending funds on written materials was wasteful in this context. Similarly, Webster et al (2003) tested an antenatal intervention aimed at reducing the incidence of postnatal depression but found that the intervention conferred no benefit on those receiving it, so other methods were proposed.

Validation of other common interventions, such as the use of pressure sore risk assessment scales and 'routine' postoperative observations, is desperately needed if nursing is to embrace a truly evidence-based culture. A useful first step would be to identify the most frequent nursing interventions and to conduct reviews of available evidence on these topics. Interventions for which there is no high-quality supporting evidence could provide a list of research priorities for state and federal bodies that fund nursing research. At present funding is ad hoc, small in scale and rarely supports large trials, which would provide the evidence needed to confirm that our interventions indeed 'do good'. We await with interest the results of such a trial currently underway in Britain. The trial is focusing on pressure relieving support surfaces for the reduction of pressure ulcers (Nelson et al 2003). This is an area where a great deal of money has been spent on such products without any evidence that they provide any benefit over existing surfaces.

However, as we suggested earlier, not all research questions are open to investigation using a randomised controlled trial.

2.3.2 Frequency questions: What is the prevalence of the problem?

One of the problems with randomised controlled trials is that they are complex to organise and conduct. They are also difficult to carry out without substantial funding. So, before investing time on such a research project, we need to ask one very essential question. Is the problem important? To determine this we may ask some subsidiary questions, such as how often does the problem occur? Does it affect a particular client group? What is the cost to the organisation? Finding evidence to answer these types of questions requires the use of techniques included under a general term of 'surveys'. These may include censuses of populations, market research studies, epidemiological studies, opinion polls, satisfaction surveys and so forth.

Surveys are usually conducted for the purpose of making descriptive statements about some population, and discovering the distribution of certain traits, attributes or disease. If we return to our example of silver sulphadiazine we may wish to find evidence about the number and type of burns that are treated at the hospital. We may also want to know how many of these burns are treated as inpatients and how many are treated as outpatients. Additional questions may include types of dressings currently used, the cost of such dressings, length of hospital stay, and the amount of nursing time spent applying and removing dressings. All of these questions are frequency questions and may be answered using the methods listed in Table 2.1. For example, a random sample of patient records may be selected, using a table of random numbers, to discover the proportion of partial to full thickness burns treated in a particular period. However, the evidence would be more accurate if a prospective, purposefully designed survey form was developed to elicit the specific information required by the researchers. Information could then be collected from a consecutive sample (all patients admitted to the burns unit) over a specified period of time. A cross-sectional survey, prevalence study or census would be used if we wanted to know how many patients on a particular day were in the hospital (or in a number of hospitals) with burn injuries.

Information (evidence) derived from the answers to frequency questions is important for building up a picture of a particular service or practice. They are vital for understanding the extent of a problem, and for determining whether or not it is worthwhile pursuing other types of research in the area. For example, if our survey revealed that a new product 'bioderm' was being used increasingly in the area but cost six times more than silver sulphadiazine, we may wish to conduct a randomised controlled trial to investigate if the new product was effective. We would want to ensure that the additional expenditure had positive benefits (e.g. reducing length of stay or improving cosmetic results).

2.3.3 Diagnosis questions: Does this person have the problem?

When looking for evidence or designing a study to answer a diagnosis question there are two primary study types, which are used for different purposes. The first relates to the use of a test (e.g. the Edinburgh Postnatal Depression Scale or EPDS) as a case-finding instrument. Our question may be: 'Should we be using the Edinburgh Postnatal Depression Scale in child-health centres as a routine screen to detect postnatal depression?'

In this case the correct approach would be to screen a consecutive sample of women at a particular time with the EPDS and compare the proportion of 'cases' identified using the screening instrument with a 'gold standard', in this instance, the DSM–IV criteria for major depression. It is important in such studies that the sensitivity, specificity and positive and negative predictive values of the case-finding screen are presented along with estimates of the 95% confidence intervals, so that the accuracy and usefulness of the screen may be evaluated (see, for example, Garcia-Esteve 2003, Garcia-Esteve et al 2003). Another illustration from our burns patient could be: 'How accurate is the presence of redness and purulent exudate in diagnosing wound infection?' In this case the gold standard would be a positive wound culture.

However, if our question related to the ability of population screening to predict the occurrence of a disease, we would need to use a randomised controlled trial in which outcomes from those screened were compared with those who were not screened. Examples of this approach include determining whether screening for colorectal cancer using a faecal occult blood test reduces colorectal cancer or whether breast cancer screening decreases deaths from breast cancer.

In the first example, a systematic review of all randomised controlled trials has shown the benefit of screening on mortality (Towler et al 2000) but, in the second example, research results remain inconsistent (Green & Taplin 2003). A useful discussion on evaluating diagnostic or screening tests can be found in the *British Medical Journal's* 'how to read a paper' series (Greenhalgh 1997a).

2.3.4 Prognosis/aetiology/harm questions: Who will get the problem, or what caused the problem?

When allocating scarce resources we may want to target a group of individuals who are most likely to develop a particular problem or suffer a particular injury. The question may be: 'Which patients are most likely to develop a wound infection?' Or 'What are the risk factors for breast cancer?' Or 'Which patients are most likely to develop a pressure ulcer?' The ideal evidence for this type of question comes from studying a group of people, a cohort, over time (e.g. all patients admitted with partial to full thickness burns, or a representative sample of all women over the age of 30, or a sample of all patients admitted to hospital during a defined period of time). At the beginning of the study, none of the cohort will have the problem or outcome (wound infection, breast cancer or pressure ulcer), but will have been exposed to one or more of the risks that may lead to its development.

The follow-up period will vary with the type of question asked. Sometimes the observation period may be decades, particularly if the question relates to risk factors associated with the development of a rare disease. There are many instances of studies that have utilised this type of evidence, which may be of interest to nurses (e.g. burnout and attrition among nurses, the relationship between night shift and colorectal cancer, and the incidence of peripheral intravenous therapy-related phlebitis (Deary et al 2003, Schernhammer et al 2003, White 2001)).

Another acceptable way to answer questions about the association between particular risk factors and development of a disease or adverse outcome is to use a case-controlled design. Compared to cohort studies, case-controlled studies are easier and cheaper to conduct, and are useful when a condition is rare. In contrast with cohort studies, the case-controlled method begins with a group of individuals with the disease of interest and a 'matched' group of individuals without the disease. Exposure to various risk factors is measured and compared between groups. For example, risk factors for breast cancer were compared using this method by Adebamowo and Adekunle (1999). Risks were identified as older age at first pregnancy and first lactation, and a higher mean number of pregnancies. The investigators also found that those with the condition had lactated less often, had used contraceptives and abused alcohol.

If we compare results from this study with findings from one of the largest cohort studies ever conducted we would note some similarities and some differences. Risks for breast cancer identified using data from the US Nurses Health Study included early age at menarche, nulliparity, having a history of benign breast disease, family history of breast cancer, the use of unopposed postmenopausal oestrogen, and 10 years of use of oestrogen plus progestin and alcohol use (Colditz & Rosner 2000).

Using results from these two studies, both reporting on risk factors associated with breast cancer, shows that data from case-controlled studies needs to be interpreted with caution. This is because data related to major risk factors may not be available, especially if a retrospective design has been used. Laupacis et al (1994) have written a useful paper, which explores these concepts in more detail (Laupacis et al 1994).

2.3.5 Phenomena questions: What are the phenomena or problems?

Phenomena questions rank highly for nurses. We want to have a direct sense of what is 'going on' for people in our care so that we can respond appropriately to their needs. Questions such as 'How do parents feel when their child is diagnosed with juvenile diabetes?', 'What are the needs of new residents in an aged care facility?' and 'What are the social and financial consequences of a diagnosis of HIV?' are examples of phenomena questions. Qualitative data-collection methods, such as in-depth interviews, focus groups or participant observation, are appropriate for answering such questions. These are methods that are concerned with generating knowledge about meaning and discovery. They are used to create theories, which may be tested using other research methods, such as surveys of large populations. Other chapters will deal with qualitative methods in more detail. In this section we are interested in whether or not the evidence from such studies may be confidently incorporated into practice.

Assessing the standard of qualitative research requires consideration of broad areas such as the effect of the interviewer (Richards & Emslie 2000), the sampling processes used and the interpretation of data. Each of these areas is open to bias and may affect the validity and, consequently, the significance and applicability of study results. Coming to terms with some of these issues has led to a great deal of effort and ongoing debate in recent years. On the one hand, attempts to develop criteria or checklists for assessing qualitative research have been proposed (Greenhalgh & Taylor 1997, Hoddinott & Pill 1997, Horsburgh 2003, Malterud 2001, Morse 2003, Whittemore et al 2001).

Arguments supporting such lists include the need for clear, systematic and reproducible methods (Greenhalgh & Taylor 1997, Hoddinott & Pill 1997), the development of assessment criteria that are specific to qualitative research (Horsburgh 2003) and the need to make it easier for 'consumers of qualitative research to critique findings in a meaningful way' (Whittemore et al 2001). However, such lists have been treated with caution by others who believe they are overprescriptive and that adherence to them has more to do with securing grant funding and publication than improving rigour (Barbour 2001, Barbour & Barbour 2003). Williams (2001) agrees and suggests that documenting reflection on the research question, the role of the investigator and his or her impact on the setting may help to fill in checklist gaps.

One of the main reasons for attempting to establish a coherent and agreed-upon set of criteria for evaluating qualitative research is to facilitate systematic reviews of papers that have addressed similar subject matter (Barbour & Barbour 2003). For example, a number of authors have addressed the question about how women experience a diagnosis of breast cancer and the subsequent treatment. Themes that have emerged include relying on prayer, avoiding negative people, developing a positive attitude, having a will to live and receiving support from family and friends (Henderson et al 2003); difficulty of living in uncertainty and of maintaining and regaining normalcy (Lam & Fielding 2003); body appearance, social support, health activism, menopause and learning to live with a chronic illness (Wilmoth & Sanders 2001); encountering darkness, converting darkness, encountering light and reflecting light (Taylor 2000); and experience trajectory, femininity and spirituality (Lackey et al 2001). Given the variety (and believability) of all of these themes, it is difficult to know how any checklist would assist in synthesising findings in any systematic way without, as Sandelowski et al (1997) put it, losing the integrity of individual studies.

Another problem in validating evidence from qualitative studies, using checklists, is that there does not appear to be any agreed-upon format. For example, Greenhalgh and Taylor (1997:741–3) have proposed 'ground rules' in the form of nine questions for evaluating qualitative research papers:

1. Did the paper describe an important clinical problem addressed via a clearly formulated question?
2. Was a qualitative approach appropriate?
3. How were the setting and the subjects selected?
4. What was the researcher's perspective and was this taken into account?
5. What methods did the researcher use for collecting data, and are these described in enough detail?
6. What methods did the researcher use to analyse the data, and what quality control measures were implemented?
7. Are the results credible, and, if so, are they clinically important?
8. What conclusions were drawn and are they justified by the results?
9. Are the results transferable to other clinical settings?

Quite a different approach to assessing validity of research findings has been put forward by Whittemore et al (2001) who suggest several evaluation techniques including 'design considerations' (e.g. sampling decisions, giving voice, employing triangulation), 'data generating' (e.g. demonstrating prolonged engagement, providing verbatim transcription, demonstrating saturation), 'analytic' (e.g. articulating data decision-analysis decisions, using computer programs, exploring rival explanations) and 'presentation' (e.g. providing an audit trail, acknowledging the researchers' perspective).

In an Australian context, the Joanna Briggs Institute (JBI) has adopted the FAME scale developed by Alan Pearson to evaluate the Feasibility, Appropriateness, Meaningfulness and Effectiveness of results of qualitative studies (JBI 2003). (See Ch 6.) However, Janet Morse (Morse 2003) has produced the most complex 'list' or series of questions, which were developed to assist those who have knowledge of qualitative methods to evaluate qualitative research proposals (Table 2.3). Many of these components could also be utilised when assessing published findings from a qualitative study. In short, evidence from qualitative studies, as with all research approaches, may provide useful information for nurses as long as the methods have been rigorous and the analysis thorough and well documented.

Table 2.3 Dimensions of evaluation criteria according to components of the proposal

Component of the proposal	Relevance	Rigour	Feasibility
1. Problem/question	A fascinating topic? Important to substantive area? Significant contribution to discipline topic and practice?	Literature review comprehensive? Synthesised? Philosophical framework identified? Analysis of concepts and theories? Use of a theoretical context? Use of a skeletal framework or scaffold?	Doable? Appropriate scope?

(continued)

Component of the proposal	Relevance	Rigour	Feasibility

2. Investigator capability	Legitimacy:
	  Able to evaluate field?
	  Able to recognise new knowledge?
	  Able to distinguish between normative and extraordinary?
		Skill:
		  Necessary experience with methods?
		  Versatile and knowledgable?
		  Able to practise reflexivity?
			Competence:
			  Necessary professional qualifications for access?
			  Adequate track record?
			  Personal characteristics for fieldwork?

3. Proposed methods	Pertinent/relevant to phenomenon? Theoretical drive?	Appropriate to question and research goal? Adequately described? Evidence of adhering to methodological assumptions? Flexibility evident?	Doable? Acceptable to participants? Appropriate context?
4. Selection of research context	Participants will provide information? (Maximise bias) Relevant to problem? (Theoretically selected) Relevant to question?	Appropriate? Maximises phenomenon? Adequate for saturation? Sample theoretically driven?	Participants feasible and accessible? Context receptive?
5. Design	Methods/strategies current and well justified?	When appropriate, permits comparison? Exploration over time? Degree of abstraction/level of explanation sought? Multiple/mixed method design?	Reconsider scope of inquiry?
6. Analytic plans	Methods will produce results in necessary form? Adequate outcome? Plans for transference/ application/ generalisability?	Proposed use of prior knowledge appropriate?	Informed/experienced investigator team?
7. Time/duration of project	Consider the stability of the phenomena studied: will it be changed/dissipated by the time the researcher reaches this point (e.g. the aftermath of a disaster)?	Time adequate for getting close to participants? Eliciting quality data? Flexibility in design? Reflection during analysis? Returning to the literature? Developing results theoretically?	Reconsider adequacy of investigator time commitment—project doable? Adequate time for 'getting in'? For saturating data? For conceptualising? For writing? For contingencies?
8. Budget	Appropriate allowance for reciprocity? Allows for dissemination/ application of results?	Adequate, considering the complexity of the project?	Adequate staff? Appropriately trained and experienced?

Component of the proposal	Relevance	Rigour	Feasibility
9. Human subjects	As proposed, no participant violations?	Feasible design as proposed? (If not feasible as proposed, will modifications affect rigour?)	Feasible setting? Permissions? Participants' safety? Researchers' safety?
10. Dissemination/ application	Plans practical?	Plans outlined?	Plans for dissemination and application doable?
11. Anticipated product: fit to existing knowledge and praxis	Usefulness?	Quality?	Applicability?

Source: Morse 2003:838–9.

2.4 Conclusion

In this chapter we have been concerned with the types of questions nurses may ask to guide their practice and have emphasised the importance of using the correct study methods to answer those questions. We have noted that many nursing interventions do not have any scientific evidence of effectiveness and suggested a way forward, which involves targeting funds for nursing research into investigations of high-frequency nursing interventions for which there is limited evidence of effect.

2.5 Discussion questions

1. Describe three patient-centred issues you have encountered recently and turn them into questions. What types of questions are they?
2. For each of the questions, describe the types of study you would search for to find an answer to your question.
3. The National Health and Medical Research Council (NHMRC) has produced 'Levels of evidence' tables. They are only useful for evaluating particular study types. What types of studies are these?
4. Discuss the issues that are associated with attempting to 'synthesise' data from qualitative studies.

2.6 References

Adebamowo C A, Adekunle O O 1999 Case-controlled study of the epidemiological risk factors for breast cancer in Nigeria. *British Journal of Surgery* 86:665–8.

Australian Government 1997 *Health and Family Services Portfolio Budget Statements 1997–98*. Commonwealth of Australia, Canberra.

Barbour R S 2001 Checklists for improving rigour in qualitative research: a case of the tail wagging the dog? *British Medical Journal* 322:1115–17.

Barbour R S, Barbour M 2003 Evaluating and synthesizing qualitative research: the need to develop a distinctive approach. *Journal of Evaluation in Clinical Practice* 9:179–86.

Begg C, Cho M, Eastwood S et al 1996 Improving the quality of reporting of randomized controlled trials. *JAMA: Journal of the American Medical Association* 276(8):637–9.

Brassey J, Elwyn G, Price C, Kinnersley P 2001 Just in time information for clinicians: a questionnaire evaluation of the ATTRACT project. *British Medical Journal* 322:529–30.

Colditz G A, Rosner B 2000 Cumulative risk of breast cancer to age 70 years according to risk factor status: data from the Nurses' Health Study. *American Journal of Epidemiology* 152(10):950–64.

Deary I J, Watson R, Hogston R 2003 A longitudinal cohort study of burnout and attrition in nursing students. *Journal of Advanced Nursing* 43:71–81.

Foxcroft D 2003 Organisational infrastructures to promote evidence based nursing practice. *Cochrane Database of Systematic Reviews* 4:CD002212.

Garcia-Esteve L, Ascaso C, Ojuel J, Navarro P 2003 Validation of the Edinburgh Postnatal Depression Scale (EPDS) in Spanish mothers. *Journal of Affective Disorders* 75:71–6.

Gould D, James T, Tarpey A et al 2000 Intervention studies to reduce the prevalence and incidence of pressure sores: a literature review. *Journal of Clinical Nursing* 9(2):163–77.

Green B B, Taplin S H 2003 Breast cancer screening controversies. *Journal of the American Board of Family Practice* 16:233–41.

Greenhalgh T 1997a How to read a paper. Papers that report diagnostic or screening tests. *British Medical Journal* 315:540–3.

Greenhalgh T 1997b Papers that summarise other papers (systematic reviews and meta-analyses). *British Medical Journal* 315:672–5.

Greenhalgh T, Taylor R 1997 Papers that go beyond numbers (qualitative research). *British Medical Journal* 315:740–3.

Henderson P D, Gore S V, Davis B L, Condon E H 2003 African-American women coping with breast cancer: a qualitative analysis. *Oncology Nursing Forum* 30:641–7.

Hicks C 1998 Barriers to evidence-based care in nursing: historical legacies and conflicting cultures. *Health Services Management Research* 11:137–47.

Hoddinott P, Pill R 1997 A review of recently published qualitative research in general practice. More methodological questions than answers? *Family Practice* 14:313–19.

Horsburgh D 2003 Evaluation of qualitative research. *Journal of Clinical Nursing* 12(2):307–12.

Joanna Briggs Institute (JBI) 2003 About the institute. Available at www.joannabriggs.edu.au/about/history.php.

Kinley H, Czoski-Murray C, George S et al 2002 Effectiveness of appropriately trained nurses in preoperative assessment: randomised controlled equivalence/non-inferiority trial. *British Medical Journal* 325:1323.

Lackey N R, Gates M F, Brown G 2001 African-American women's experiences with the initial discovery, diagnosis, and treatment of breast cancer. *Oncology Nursing Forum* 28:519–27.

Lam W W T, Fielding R 2003 The evolving experience of illness for Chinese women with breast cancer: a qualitative study. *Psycho-Oncology* 12:127–40.

Laupacis A, Wells G, Richardson W S, Tugwell P 1994 Users' guides to the medical literature. V. How to use an article about prognosis. Evidence-Based Medicine Working Group. *JAMA: Journal of the American Medical Association* 272:234–7.

Malterud K 2001 Qualitative research: standards, challenges, and guidelines. *Lancet* 358:483–8.

Moher D, Schulz K F, Altman D G 2003 The CONSORT statement: revised recommendations for improving the quality of reports of parallel-group randomised trials. *Clinical Oral Investigations* 7:2–7.

Moore K H, O'Sullivan R J, Simons A et al 2003 Randomised controlled trial of nurse continence advisor therapy compared with standard urogynaecology regimen for conservative incontinence treatment: efficacy, costs and two year follow up. *British Journal of Gynaecology* 110:649–57.

Moore L, Campbell R, Whelan A et al 2002 Self-help smoking cessation in pregnancy: cluster randomised controlled trial. *British Medical Journal* 325:1383.

Morse J M 2003 A review committee's guide for evaluating qualitative proposals. *Qualitative Health Research* 13:833–51.

National Health and Medical Research Council (NHMRC) 1999 *A guide to the development, implementation and evaluation of clinical practice guidelines*, Appendix B, p 56. Australian Government Publishing Service, Canberra.

Nelson E A, Nixon J, Mason S et al 2003 A nurse-led randomised trial of pressure-relieving support surfaces. *Professional Nurse* 18:513–16.

NSW Health 2000 *Strategic directions for health 2000–05*. NSW Health Department, Sydney.

Pinnock H, Bawden R, Proctor S et al 2003 Accessibility, acceptability, and effectiveness in primary care of routine telephone review of asthma: pragmatic, randomised controlled trial. *British Medical Journal* 326:477–9.

Pravikoff D S, Donaldson N E 2001 Online journals: access and support for evidence-based practice. AACN. *Clinical Issues* 12:588–96.

Queensland Health 2003a Getting your clinical question ready for searching, in *Clinician Development Program Education Service Facilitator Kit*. Queensland Health, Brisbane.

Queensland Health 2003b *Queensland Health strategic plan 2003–07*. Queensland Health, Brisbane.

Richards H, Emslie C 2000 The 'doctor' or the 'girl from the University'? Considering the influence of professional roles on qualitative interviewing. *Family Practice* 17:71–5.

Sandelowski M, Docherty S, Emden C 1997 Focus on qualitative methods. Qualitative metasynthesis: issues and techniques. *Research in Nursing and Health* 20:365–71.

Schernhammer E S, Laden F, Speizer F E et al 2003. Night-shift work and risk of colorectal cancer in the nurses' health study. *Journal of the National Cancer Institute* 95:825–8.

Taylor E J 2000 Transformation of tragedy among women surviving breast cancer. *Oncology Nursing Forum* 27:781–8.

Towler B P, Irwig L, Glasziou P et al 2000 Screening for colorectal cancer using the faecal occult blood test, hemoccult. *Cochrane Database Systematic Reviews* CD001216.

Webster J, Linnane J, Roberts J et al 2003 IDentify, Educate and Alert (IDEA) trial: an intervention to reduce postnatal depression. *British Journal of Obstetrics and Gynaecology* 110:842–6.

White S A 2001 Peripheral intravenous therapy-related phlebitis rates in an adult population. *Journal of Intravenous Nursing* 24:19–24.

Whittemore R, Chase S K, Mandle C L 2001 Validity in qualitative research. *Qualitative Health Research* 11:522–37.

Williams B 2001 Checklists for improving rigour in qualitative research. Including personal reflections might help. *British Medical Journal* 323:515.

Wilmoth M C, Sanders L D 2001 Accept me for myself: African-American women's issues after breast cancer. *Oncology Nursing Forum* 28:875–9.

chapter ③

Quantitative research designs

Diana Battistutta and Jan McDowell

3.1 Learning objectives

After reading this chapter, you should be able to:

1. *describe the philosophical underpinnings of quantitative research*
2. *describe the elements that define the ideal quantitative research design*
3. *analyse the reasons why less-than-ideal quantitative research design is often implemented, and adequate, and*
4. *analyse how different quantitative research designs influence the credibility of evidence.*

3.2 Introduction

Many of the questions arising in nursing practice revolve around the effectiveness and acceptability of current interventions or practices—to patients, to staff, or to management. The requirement for continuous practice improvement thus mandates the collection of credible evidence to support practice changes. Credible evidence captures current reality and provides objective information to support an argument for change in that reality. Both qualitative and quantitative research may do this, although the perspectives from which the research is approached are very different, as suggested by the introduction in Chapter 2 and as you will see from reading and comparing Chapters 3 and 4.

Our knowledge is acquired from a wide variety of sources—some anecdotal (e.g. a friend's recent experience with acute appendicitis), and some more formal (e.g. published hospital reports about adverse events from appendicectomies performed in the previous year). We often subconsciously evaluate the quality of this information for credibility as a source of evidence. Some sources of information are more objective than others (e.g. individuals' experiences posted on their personal web page compared to newspaper reports compared to medical journal articles on surgical complications of an appendicectomy). Quantitative research design is a planning exercise by which maximum objectivity and consistency are brought to every facet of the evidence-gathering process so that research results are as credible and generalisable as possible.

The purpose of this chapter is to provide an overview of the quantitative research process, its philosophical underpinnings, and to describe particular quantitative designs that inform the framework for projects undertaken by nurse researchers and health researchers more generally. No design is perfect, and a knowledge of the strengths and weaknesses of the various designs will help in assessing the quality of evidence with which we are confronted on a daily basis.

3.3 Philosophical underpinnings of quantitative research

There are several paradigms (views or models) of thinking about how the world works. In health research in general, there are two main paradigms under which research is designed: the *naturalistic* paradigm and the *positivist* paradigm.

3.3.1 The naturalistic and positivist paradigms

The naturalistic paradigm emphasises the importance of the whole experience, seeking patterns or themes in participants' descriptions of events/processes. The researcher has no preconceived views of what to expect of the information to be collected in the course of the research, and there is an emphasis on allowing individuals' experiences to shape the final conclusions or themes to arise from the research. This perspective was introduced in Chapter 2 and will be detailed in Chapter 4. It is the paradigm under which qualitative research is undertaken.

In contrast, the positivist paradigm emphasises one or several very well-defined aspects of the whole experience, predetermined by the researcher. These aspects may be derived from clinical experience, current research literature, or prior qualitative research, which has identified particular questions that need addressing in detail. Research under this paradigm involves precise measurement of very specific aspects, and is usually aimed at verifying or disproving the researcher's prespecified expectations. As such, mainly quantitative data are collected.

Most researchers working under a positivist paradigm wish to infer their results beyond the group being studied. Practice or policy change would not ensue unless the collected evidence for change was generalisable to wider practice. The degree to which such inference (generalisation) is possible depends on the type and quality of the research design implemented to answer the research question. The process of inference is integral to quantitative research design, and is underpinned by the concept of scientific deduction.

3.3.2 Logical reasoning: inductive and deductive thinking under a positivist paradigm

Quantitative research methodology evolved from the philosophies of mathematics and science. These philosophies gained credence during the sixteenth century following a long intellectual battle between the Church and emerging scientists who put forward theories for explaining and predicting occurrences in the natural world. This period in the development of science was known as the beginning of the Enlightenment. Francis Bacon (1561–1626) was an influential scientist at this time and argued that the process of undertaking science involved four logical steps:

1. observing or experiencing an event
2. formulating an hypothesis about that event
3. conducting an experiment to test the hypothesis, and
4. drawing a conclusion based on whether the hypothesis is supported or not.

Over time these steps have been embraced as the basis of a scientific method that assists researchers to organise their thought processes in a rational and systematic manner.

The philosophy of science advanced during four centuries of Enlightenment. Two scientists who were particularly influential during that time were Isaac Newton (1642–1727) and Auguste Comte (1798–1857). It is now legendary that Newton was sitting under an apple tree one day and an apple fell on his head. This auspicious event prompted Newton to use the scientific method proposed by Bacon to test out his theory on gravity. The outcome was the Universal Law of Gravitation. Comte's scientific endeavours focused on examining and explaining the sociological world. Comte proposed that the objective when acquiring scientific knowledge is simply to describe an unusual or significant occurrence without questioning whether it exists or not. He argued that hierarchical methods of scientific inquiry, such as those used in hard science by Bacon and Newton, were equally applicable when investigating aspects of society. Comte is recognised as the founder of Positivism, a scientific movement that believes all human knowledge is based on observation of natural events.

The most influential scientific philosophy at the beginning of the twentieth century was an extension of Comte's work known as Logical Positivism (sometimes called Logical Empiricism). This movement began in Vienna during the 1920s with discussions among a group of scientists about current thinking on logic. As an outcome of those discussions the group, known as the Vienna Circle, argued that there are only two sources of knowledge: logical reasoning and empirical experience. According to the Circle, logical reasoning is derived from *a priori* knowledge (e.g. if today is Monday then today is not Friday), whereas empirical experience is based on *a posteriori* knowledge (e.g. humans tend to dislike pain).

Logical reasoning is based on the processes of induction and deduction. Inductive reasoning progresses from the particular to the general. That is, particulars are observed (e.g. Mary has red hair; Mary is bad-tempered) and a generalisation is made (e.g. all red-haired people are bad-tempered). From experience we would know that this is not true. Therefore, care must be taken with generalisations from inductive reasoning. In contrast, the deductive process progresses from the general to the particular. That is, a generalisation is made (e.g. every horse has four legs) and particulars are observed (e.g. no horse has two legs). A conclusion is made (therefore, horses always have four legs). It is reasonable to assume that this argument is true. However, if the deductive process is applied in a different context (e.g. all sovereigns are worth 20 shillings; the Queen is a sovereign; therefore, the Queen is worth 20 shillings), the conclusion may be inaccurate.

Karl Popper (1902–94), a member of the Vienna Circle as a young scientist, became a strong critic of the inductive and, to a certain extent, deductive methods of reasoning. Popper strove to address the question 'What reason have we for supposing any scientific theory to be true?' (Adams & Dyson 2003:200). Popper argued that it is impossible to positively verify a universal scientific theory. Based on this argument he proposed the Popperian Theory of Falsification. That is, it doesn't matter how many instances of a particular are observed, it is impossible to confirm a hypothesis. However, it is possible to refute a hypothesis with only one observation. Therefore, one can only disprove a universal theory. Popper cautions, however, that a theory should only be rejected when there is a better theory derived through objective growth of knowledge (Andersson 1994).

Logical Positivism has played a very important role in the development of contemporary scientific philosophy. Most modern social research using quantitative research design involves inductive and deductive reasoning processes at some point. That is, a research project may begin as an open-ended exploration of a particular outcome (inductive reasoning), and then narrow in focus to test out a hypothesis (deductive reasoning). Finally, the research may be underpinned by the Theory of Falsification in which the researcher aims to demonstrate the exception, and disprove a hypothesis.

The Theory of Falsification is reflected in scientific hypothesis testing that is a part of most quantitative research.

3.4 The quantitative research process

Inferential quantitative research proceeds on the basis that there is a status quo (null hypothesis) that the researcher believes may be improved (alternate hypothesis). The current state is the 'truth' until a new 'truth' takes its place. Investment in research mainly proceeds on the premise that the alternate hypothesis is more likely (why should resources be wasted on reproving the status quo?). Based on the Theory of Falsification, it takes only one exception to disprove the null hypothesis. Hence, in the quantitative research process, information is collected to provide as much objective evidence as possible against the null, such that it can be concluded that the new state, expressed in the alternate hypothesis, is more likely to be the truth.

Most quantitative research aims to compare an outcome across groups, over time, or has both elements incorporated. The null hypothesis in the first example would be that there are no differences in outcome across the groups; the alternate hypothesis would be that at least one group demonstrates substantially different outcomes.

Having established the scientific hypothesis requiring testing, the quantitative research process consists typically of the following steps:
1. *Design:*
   —selecting a comprehensive list of subjects (sampling frame) who are eligible to participate
   —determining a sampling strategy to optimise representative participation of a subgroup (this is to ensure generalisability of results)
   —defining appropriate comparison groups
   —identifying measurement tools (questionnaires, instruments) to measure study outcomes, and
   —establishing the quality of the measurement tools in terms of measurement validity and reproducibility or reliability.

2. *Data collection:*
   —piloting planned data-collection procedures and refining if necessary, and
   —collecting the main data.
3. *Hypothesis testing:*
   —statistical analysis to test the scientific hypothesis
   —considering (analytically) the potential for competing explanations of the result, and
   —reporting on the results (e.g. if the null hypothesis cannot be rejected based on the collected data, there is no change to policy or practice).

Of course, despite best efforts, imperfections may surface in any aspect of the research process. Biased procedures may distort the quantitative measurements, participants may not be representative of the wider pool, and comparison groups may become privy to each others' intervention and change their behaviour accordingly. Imperfections in research are to be expected, but need to be identified and reviewed critically for their impact on the results.

Remembering that the results will choose the null or alternate hypothesis as the most likely explanation for the collected data, there are two potential types of inferential error:
1. A type I error is considered the most serious. This occurs where the alternate hypothesis is mistakenly accepted over the null hypothesis, and a difference across groups (e.g. over time) is mistakenly reported.
2. A type II error is considered less serious. This occurs where the alternate hypothesis is not accepted over the null hypothesis when it should be, and a real difference is discounted.

To avoid incorrect conclusions from the research, the ideal quantitative research design will control all possible known sources of bias that may eventuate in the context of that research.

Some designs permit more control than others, although because health research is usually of free-living human beings in whom minimal manipulation is ethically permitted, and in whom a range of health outcomes develop over years rather than weeks or months, a variety of quantitative research designs have developed to accommodate the associated restrictions. The final choice of design is based on the type of hypothesis being tested, practical resources available, and ethical considerations. While all designs consider all of the above-listed elements, variations have ramifications for the relative quality of the resulting evidence. Having knowledge of the most common quantitative research designs, in particular their strengths and weaknesses, is important in reviewing research evidence and research literature for credibility.

3.5 The ideal quantitative research design

Ideally, all research would be undertaken under highly controlled experimental conditions such as in the laboratory, where, with one exception, nothing varies (i.e. genetically similar animals exposed to environmentally similar physical and psychological conditions). The exception is the intervention in which the scientist is interested. If all else is equal (by design), then any variation across groups is causally due to the intervention. The perfect experiment is the only design in which statements of causal relationship may be made with confidence. Quantitative research designs for health research attempt to mimic this level of control as best they can. The ability to attribute causality is the highest form of research evidence available (e.g. a certain drug causes lipid lowering because all else was held constant in the design).

Many quantitative research designs will result only in reports of association due to the limiting features of the design falling short of attributing causality to the relationship (e.g. a certain drug is associated with lipid lowering, but all was not held equal in design, and the result may be a spurious one due to the drug group having lower lipid levels before intervention).

Practically speaking, the ideal quantitative design for health research is the experimental design. Although the nomenclature is similar, the elements of an 'experiment' when dealing with free-living humans are different from those of the 'true' experiment in a laboratory. However, there is a strong attempt to create an 'all else equal' environment.

3.5.1 Experimental studies

There are three characteristics of experimental study design:
- they involve comparison groups with different *interventions* (or manipulation)
- there is a *control* group, and
- participants are allocated randomly (i.e. *randomisation*).

Experimental designs always involve comparison groups with different experimental conditions or *interventions*. There may be two or more groups. The researcher determines what interventions are to be allocated and there is usually a finite and relatively small number (e.g. half of all participants in a study of effective pain relief are allocated to using protocol A and the other half to protocol B).

Control specifically refers to the allocation of one of the comparison groups to a *control group* status. Subjects in this group get no intervention, and experience standard care or the 'usual' experience, or a placebo of some sort. With data on a control group, it is possible to determine the excess effect of the intervention over and above any natural changes that would have occurred. This strengthens the ability of the researcher to place a *causal* interpretation on the results.

Random allocation of participants to intervention groups means that there is an equal chance of a subject being allocated to any one of the interventions. This minimises the possibility that the comparison groups are unbalanced in any way. It is the most efficient way of ensuring that *all* characteristics are equally represented in all comparison (intervention) groups, so that we can maximise the chance of truly saying 'all else equal'. Randomisation takes the allocation of subjects to groups out of the hands of the researcher and submits it to chance.

The experimental design is the most controlled research design, and, as such, has the least potential of all study designs to produce biased conclusions. However, precisely due to the amount of control and manipulation that is inherent in experimental study designs, it is obvious that they are very artificial situations, not reflecting the real world. This sometimes makes them a completely inappropriate design for particular research questions. Often to achieve this degree of control, there is substantial restriction of eligibility of study subjects, to the point where generalisability is compromised. For example, while we may be able to say that drug A was an effective lipid-lowering drug, we may have had to restrict our study to healthy males under

50 years of age. What can we say about the effects of this drug on older persons, or those with heart conditions, or females? Also, under such artificial control, the intervention condition is an ideal that is usually not met in the real world. For example, while we may ask subjects to apply 1 g of sunscreen per day, no one in the real world would measure their sunscreen before application. They would apply an 'adequate' amount that might be more or less than the amount prescribed during the study.

When designing a research study, it is important to consider whether it is practical to design it as an experimental study. If so, this is the design of choice. Other designs are not as controlled and hence increase the potential for bias in the results. However, often experiments are not possible, and a 'lesser' quality study design will be the design of choice.

3.5.2 Sources of error and bias

Because we cannot perfectly control the real world in which research is performed, there is always the potential for error to be introduced at any level in the research design or execution process. There are two types of error: *random* (or chance) error and systematic error (or *bias*). Random error is unpredictable in direction—sometimes being an overestimation, sometimes an underestimation, of the true measurement. It occurs to equal degrees across comparison groups. While random error introduces 'noise' into measurements, it does not distort the comparison of intervention and control group differences—neither will a systematic error applied equally across all comparison groups. The measurements will be distorted, but equally so in all groups. Serious bias is introduced when measurements or other critical study procedures are differentially applied across comparison groups, resulting in a dilution or exaggeration of the comparison between intervention and control groups.

There are several sources of potential bias in research. These are:
1. *Selection bias*, which leads to an unrepresentative group of participants. This has ramifications for the interpretation (*generalisability*) of research results, as self-selected samples tend to be more motivated, and, in health research, this may be due to other health issues.
2. *Confounding*, which is a bias introduced when comparison groups have different underlying characteristics, such that there are competing explanations for any group differences. A classic confounding variable in health research is age, a competing explanation for many health relationships, due to it being a marker variable for physiological deterioration associated with most health issues.
3. *Information bias*, which is where measurements are taken differently within the study comparison groups (e.g. different personnel achieving different levels of rapport with patients collect data in the different groups).

3.6 Less-than-ideal but practical quantitative research designs

As suggested above, there is a 'quality' continuum in the design of quantitative research studies. The most common designs implemented in nursing and health research in general include, in order from most controlled to least controlled, and hence with increasing potential to bias the resulting research:

1. *Experimental*
2. *Quasi-experimental:*
   —prepost test, and
   —post-test.
3. *Observational:*
   (a) Correlational:
      —cohort
      —case-control, and
      —cross-sectional.
   (b) Descriptive:
      —case-series, and
      —case-study.

3.6.1 Experimental designs

The design of highest quality is the *experimental* design. Unless all three elements of an experiment are present, there is potential for introducing bias into research results. Indeed, even experiments are not perfect (consider a perfectly executed experiment on a badly selected non-representative group of people—of what use are these results?). Practical advantages of 'lesser' quality designs often outweigh the risks of bias introduced by using such approaches. By choosing a less-than-ideal experiment, the resulting research is not necessarily less credible. The design planning, however, will need to incorporate checks and balances to ensure that the known potential for bias does not override the quality of such studies.

3.6.2 Quasi-experimental designs

Quasi-experimental study designs involve an intervention but do not randomise participants to an intervention group (introducing potential confounding bias), or do not have a control comparison group (excluding the estimating of a true intervention effect over and above natural change in the absence of intervention). The consequent 'drop' on the design quality scale is implied with the loss of the benefits associated with one or both features. This reduction in design quality most obviously affects the ability to imply causation from findings. However, due to the reduction in control over their design, quasi-experimental designs are flexible and often the only practical alternative. Often they do not restrict the eligibility of subjects to the same degree as a true experimental design, making the results of such studies more generalisable to the wider population. Care needs to be taken in the interpretation of results from quasi-experimental studies, but they are certainly a very popular alternative in health research.

Another quasi-experimental quantitative study design gaining popularity in the medical literature is the $n = 1$ study. This design involves only one person or observational unit with repeated measures under different conditions. Various treatments are applied to the same individual, and their response under each condition is monitored. For example, a cream for the control of eczema may be tried out on one individual. The individual acts as his or her own control, since the eczema should clear under the application of cream, and reappear in the absence of cream. If this cycle of disappearance/reappearance can be demonstrated more than once, the design has effectively shown the effectiveness of the cream.

3.6.3 Observational study designs

Further down on the quality continuum are the study designs that have no 'experimental' features whatsoever, the observational study designs. *Observational* study designs include those broadly called correlational and descriptive.

3.6.3.1 Correlational studies

Correlational study designs summarise associations between variables, usually with a view to generating hypotheses. These do not manipulate an intervention and they do not randomly allocate people to comparison groups. They are solely based on observing what happens or happened. Occasionally, they do have control groups, but not in the allocated sense of a manipulated intervention. Again, these designs, due to their total or near-total lack of control, are prone to confounding bias. Despite this, their popularity comes from the fact that they are quick and easy to execute and usually require fewer resources than the more experimental designs. A well-executed observational study can be very valuable and produce valid conclusions, although often they are used to generate hypotheses rather than definitively answer research questions. This is because it is difficult to ascribe causality to the relationships between outcome and explanatory variables, unlike in an experimental design with its inherent controls.

Although there are many variants and hybrid designs, the three most commonly used observational quantitative research designs in health research are the *cohort* study, the *case-control* study and the *cross-sectional* study designs.

A *cohort* study design is one where individuals are prospectively followed up over time. Subjects in cohort studies are selected on the basis of their membership of a particular group (e.g. all spinal injury patients with pressure sores; all nurses from the same ward). Cohort studies are *longitudinal* studies, since they involve repeated measurements over time. Outcomes of interest are defined as newly observed events forward in time (prospectively). Because the events are observed to occur after exposure, the ability to infer causality is possible, assuming 'all else being equal' can be incorporated into the design.

Cohort studies can also be retrospective, auditing records backwards in time to count events, although this is a less common design. Such designs are based on historical records that have been collected for purposes other than research. One extra potential source of bias in the data-collection process for this design therefore relates to the inconsistent quality of data recorded in these historical records.

A *case-control* study design also, and only ever, involves retrospective data collection, but the design is the inverse of the cohort study. In the above, we identify a cohort and categorise persons into comparison groups according to their exposure status. We then count events (cases) of the outcome as they develop over time. In the case-control approach, the cases with events would be identified from historical records and data collection would involve determining their prior exposures, usually over long periods of life. This procedure would be repeated in a group of identified controls, persons without the event of interest but similar in all other respects to the cases. Hence not one but two separate groups of persons are studied from two separate pools of people. This design is very popular when the event rate is slow to accumulate (e.g. rare conditions such as cancer), where a cohort study would take years to accumulate even a small number of events.

The choice of a suitable control group is tricky in the design of case-control studies. A control group must be similar in all respects to the case group, otherwise there is the chance that imbalances (confounding factors) are introduced into the comparison groups. When case groups are based in hospitals rather than population-based, the choice of control group becomes even more difficult. There is often a difficult choice between healthy non-hospital controls, or hospital-based controls, and it is not uncommon for both types of control groups to be selected in the one study design.

A *cross-sectional* study design is just that—a view of relationships at a 'slice' in time (i.e. collecting data at one time point). The most common form of the cross-sectional design is the survey, by questionnaire or interview. Relationships between variables are summarised in appropriate ways (formally known as correlation) to determine the strength of any associations. Because it is difficult in cross-sectional studies to ascribe temporal (time) order to exposures and events, these studies are prone to biases more than any other of the designs so far described. However, they are invaluable as exploratory studies aimed at generating firmer research questions.

It is possible to design a research study that comprises several cross-sectional studies over time. For example, to monitor the rate of smoking in adolescents, it would be reasonable to do a cross-sectional survey of a random sample of adolescents in each year from 2000 to 2005. The percentage of adolescents who smoke would be summarised for each year. Note that this is *not* a cohort study, even though it is counting events (smokers) over time. A cohort study would monitor the *same* adolescents over time and not a different group each time (some overlap may occur but it is still not a cohort design).

3.6.3.2 Descriptive studies

Descriptive studies are usually designed to provide basic information in the absence of knowledge. Generally, they are not meant to consider relationships between variables. For example, a study may be designed to determine the prevalence (or proportion) of the community that uses acupuncture for pain relief. Descriptive studies can be the most prone to introduced biases (mainly selection and confounding biases), due to the absence of a comparison or control group.

A *case-series* is usually done in the pioneering phase of research, when a researcher has a hunch that there may be an association between two variables, but does not have enough data to support a full research project. As much *descriptive* data as possible on a broad range of characteristics are collected on a series of like cases and common features are summarised. For example, in the 1990s there were several cases of Creutzfeldt-Jakob (CJD) disease in Britain. This condition is a very rare acute, brain-debilitating disease and the numbers of 'events' were in relatively epidemic proportions. Data were collected on the 10 or so cases that occurred close together in time, and it was determined that the common element in these cases was the exposure in their diet to bovine offal. Consumption in turn was finally linked to the transmission, from cow to human, of the agent that caused a similar brain disease in bovines.

As a question-generating design, this simple case-series was very effective. As a definitive study, there were problems. There was only a small number of cases, and there was no control group. What if people without CJD ate bovine offal as often as those with CJD, and the common characteristic was just coincidence? Having outlined the major deficiencies of the case-series as a study design, it must be stated that no other higher quality study design would be possible in such a situation due to the ethical and practical constraints.

The *case-study* is the most basic study 'design', where an individual's experience is documented in a quantitative way. This is commonly seen in medical journals where interesting, usually rare, medical cases are described. In the example above, the first event of CJD may have been written up as a case-study with all medical tests and history detailed.

3.6.3.3 Advantage of observational studies

The main advantage of observational study designs is that there is no artificial intervention on individuals, nor are subjects artificially allocated to different study groups. Subjects are observed in their 'natural' state. This is sometimes the only way that research can be done, as some variables are not subject to manipulation (consider marital status, health beliefs, medical illness, skin colour). Sometimes it is an ethical reason that precludes manipulation, in that it is unethical to withhold the usual standard of care, or to expose people to hazards to which they would not normally be exposed. Because people self-select into different groups (e.g. unhealthy people are motivated to complete surveys about health, gregarious people are more likely to be in public relations work than shy persons), there is a very real chance that characteristics of comparison groups are unbalanced, introducing confounding bias and making a valid comparison more difficult than in the experimental setting.

3.7 Conclusion

Quantitative research is characterised by postulating very specific questions based on *a priori* expectations of the results being different from the status quo. The research process involves collecting data (evidence) in as controlled and objective a manner as possible within resource and ethical limits. This evidence will be used to decide whether or not the data are more consistent with the *a priori* expectation or more so with the status quo.

Experimental designs provide the most rigorously controlled research process, permitting statements of causality to be made. This is often at the expense of generalisablity of the results due to the artificial restrictions required to optimise control. Observational study designs are more easily executed than experimental designs since interventions are not imposed on individuals. Observational designs are flexible in that they permit heterogeneous groups of participants to be involved, providing opportunities to generalise to broad target populations. Potential confounding factors are expected in such studies, leading to competing explanations for the final study results. As long as potential confounding factors are identified and measured as part of the research plan, the risks for biased conclusions can be minimised in observational studies.

It is not necessary that a research study be executed perfectly; indeed even the most rigorously designed and executed experimental study will have weaknesses. The key issue to consider is whether or not any identified weaknesses have an impact on the conclusions. If biases are noted and not discussed or accounted for, this should raise concerns about the credibility of any research study.

The checklist in Table 3.1 suggests the key design questions that help to identify potential problems. It summarises questions that you should ask each time you read a research article. If your answer is 'no' to any of the questions, when critiquing a particular article, write down *why* you think the answer is 'no'. After you have worked through the checklist, your written list of limitations will guide you when deciding whether or not you agree with the researchers' report of their work. Remember, the *aim of a critique* is to decide if the work has sufficient error or bias in the results, such that the conclusions would be different if the study did not have these errors or biases. There will be limitations in every study; the point is to determine if the limitations are sufficient to cause the conclusion the authors have reached to be incorrect.

Table 3.1 Checklist for appraising quality of published quantitative research

Question	Yes/No
1. Is there a clear statement of the aims of the study, such that a scientific hypothesis is offered or implied?	□/□
2. Are there detailed definitions of the outcome variable(s)?	□/□
3. Are there detailed definitions of the comparison to be made (over groups or time, or both)?	□/□
4. Consider the description of the target population, the sampling source and the sampling strategy. Do you think it led to a representative sample of the target population?	□/□
5. Is the study a fully experimental study design?	□/□
6. If yes, is there a table showing the success of randomisation with balanced characteristics across all comparison groups?	□/□
7. If yes, there is little risk of confounding variables having an influence on results. If no, there is a risk for potential confounding by the unbalanced variables. Have they been accounted for in the analysis by 'statistical adjustment'?	□/□
8. Are you satisfied with the quality of measurement (reproducibility, validity) of the outcome variable(s)?	□/□
9. Are there low proportions of missing data for the key variables involved in testing the hypothesis? (A lot of missing data may lead to selection bias.)	□/□
10. If a follow-up study, is the attrition rate of participants over time low? (High attrition may lead to selection bias.)	□/□
11. Were ethical issues discussed and accounted for in the design?	□/□
12. Have the results been presented in a way that corresponds to the scientific hypotheses?	□/□
13. Is the discussion of conclusions consistent with the results as presented?	□/□
14. Have the authors generalised the results to the correct target population?	□/□
15. Was the research done independently of any conflicting sources of interest (e.g. funding by a source with interest in the outcome of the study, such as a tobacco company)?	□/□

The highest level of evidence for best practice comes from formal systematic reviews of multiple experimental-level studies on the same research question. Often, there is only one opportunity to do a randomised controlled study, or no opportunity at all when ethical constraints are considered. Sometimes the intervention of interest cannot be randomised practically in a hospital setting. Objective critique of well-executed quantitative research studies can provide adequate evidence for change in practice or policy. An awareness of the potential biases introduced by research at any level is the key to assessing the value of any quantitative research.

3.8 Discussion questions

1. Would evidence collected with a quantitative research design be suitable to inform your nursing practice?
2. What types of research questions within your nursing practice would not be able to be answered with a quantitative research design?
3. What practical sources of error might be introduced during the execution of a quantitative research project in your nursing practice?
4. How would you go about designing a quantitative study to determine the relative effectiveness of acupuncture on postoperative pain relief?
5. How would you go about designing a quantitative study to determine the impact of new security measures on the incidence of verbal or physical abuse to nursing staff in the emergency department?

3.9 References

Adams I, Dyson R W 2003 *Fifty major political thinkers*. Routledge, London.
Andersson G 1994 *Criticism and the history of science*. E J Brill, Leiden, The Netherlands.
Bowling A 1997 *Research methods in health. Investigating health and health services*. Open University Press, Buckingham.
DePoy E, Gitlin L N 1998 *Introduction to research. Understanding and applying multiple strategies*. Mosby, St Louis.
Horwich P (ed) 1993 *World changes: Thomas Kuhn and the nature of science*. Massachusetts Institute of Technology, Boston.
Jenkinson C (ed) 1997 *Assessment and evaluation of health and medical care. A methods text*. Open University Press, Buckingham.
Lipton P (ed) 1995 *Theory, evidence and explanation volume 14*. Dartmouth, Aldershot.
Polit D F, Beck C T 2004 *Nursing research. Principles and methods*. Lippincott Williams & Wilkins, Philadelphia.
Popper K 2002 *Conjectures and refutations: the growth of scientific knowledge*. Routledge, London.
Schneider Z, Elliott D, LoBiondo-Wood G, Haber J 2003 *Nursing research: Methods, critical appraisal and utilisation*, 2nd edn. Elsevier (Australia), Sydney.
Sharrock W, Read R 2002 *Kuhn: philosopher of scientific revolution*. Polity Press, Cambridge.

chapter ④

Qualitative research designs

Mary FitzGerald and John Field

4.1 Learning objectives

After reading this chapter, you should be able to:

1. *discuss what constitutes 'qualitative research'*
2. *construct an argument that supports the use of qualitative evidence in a program of clinical research, and*
3. *be critically aware of your own ability to select a methodology that matches a particular clinical research question or problem.*

4.2 Introduction

The purpose of this chapter is to present qualitative research and situate it as a perspective of equal prominence, albeit for different contributions, to quantitative research in the discipline of nursing. In the other sections of this book authors draw attention to the use of evidence to support clinical practice and decisions; findings from qualitative research are a rich source of evidence.

The understandings generated from qualitative research may be used by astute clinicians to support decisions regarding the appropriateness of actions connected with health service delivery. They are a source of information that enables clinicians to relate to the personal, cultural, social and political situation in contemporary health services, and provide care that is sensitive to the needs of the individual. By extension, qualitative researchers provide information that illuminates the complexity of health service delivery, thus putting the informed clinician in a better position to make a fair assessment of particular situations and to choose actions that are most appropriate in that instance.

The methodologies most commonly employed by nursing research students are phenomenology, ethnography and grounded theory. Action research is widely used by practice developers and more recently as a means to implement and evaluate best available evidence in practice. These familiar methodologies will be described in this chapter. The methodologies employed by researchers in the large programs in North America are well reported in broader nursing literature and in particular the *Journal of Qualitative Health Research*. Each year there is a meeting of minds at the

International Qualitative Health Research Conference where many nurses gather to report on findings, but also to debate and discuss the nuances of and developments in qualitative research methodology.

4.3 What is qualitative research?

'Qualitative research', although a collective term, may create a misconception of unity. It refers in reality to a cluster of broadly divergent research methodologies. There is, as will unfold in this chapter, a range of research approaches used to guide the collection and use of qualitative data in nursing research. From any of a number of perspectives or paradigms, each with ontological and epistemological position/s, researchers collect, analyse and interpret qualitative data to present more understanding of the world and its constitutive elements.

A pragmatist may deduce that qualitative research appears to represent all that is to do with words or that is not numerical/statistical. It is, however, inaccurate to suggest that qualitative researchers deal exclusively with words. Researchers using these methodologies collect a variety of symbols to explore, reveal and re-present information that enlightens human understanding of social experiences and their meanings. Nevertheless, these researchers do share a view that texts in a variety of forms (e.g. artworks, photographs, cinema, performance, literature, biography) provide data that can be more richly illuminative of the world than statistics.

Denzin and Lincoln (1998:407), world-renowned authors on the subject of qualitative research, argue that qualitative researchers are bound together by:

> ... this centre [that] lies in the humanistic commitment of the
> qualitative researcher to study the world always from the perspective
> of the interacting individual. From this simple commitment flow the
> liberal and radical politics of qualitative research.

Their definition of qualitative research (Denzin & Lincoln 1998:408) broadly incorporates a range of disciplines, a desire to pursue understanding from a naturalistic perspective within a context that is '. . . shaped by multiple ethical and political positions . . .' and furthermore, balances the generation of knowledge through broad understanding of context and narrow analysis of the particular. This is a vantage point that suits the dominant ideology of nursing, which is focused on individualised and holistic forms of caring (Pearson et al 2004). Of course, that ideology competes in the practical world with dogmas associated with medical science and economics that appear to be most influential in the evidence-based practice (EBP) movement.

Streubert and Carpenter (1999:15) have found the following *characteristics* of qualitative researchers:

> ... a belief in multiple realities; a commitment to identifying an
> approach to understanding that supports the phenomenon studied;
> a commitment to the participant's viewpoint; the conduct of
> inquiry in a way that limits disruption of the natural context of
> the phenomena of interest; acknowledged participation of the
> researcher in the research; and the conveyance of an
> understanding of phenomena by reporting in a literary
> style rich with participant commentaries.

These ideas relate to the underlying assumptions about reality and know-ledge that are discussed and examined at a philosophical level in the ontological (being) and epistemological (knowledge) bases of research per-spectives. They are not exhaustive or universally representative of all qualitative research methodologies, but they demonstrate the link between research paradigm, research methodology and research methods that are made explicit in qualitative research studies. Denzin and Lincoln (1998:23) refer to the 'interpretive community' that provides those philosophical assumptions that form a base from which researchers set out with confidence to pursue social phenomena in particular ways.

In summary, there is not a clear definition of 'qualitative research' that does justice to its potential or complexity. However, qualitative data is relatively easy to recognise when understood as any data that is not numerical. This is a some-what limited but useful definition. Qualitative researchers embrace a range of methodologies that are underpinned by assumptions regarding the nature and generation of understanding/knowledge in the world. Typically qualitative research studies are prefaced with relatively long methodology sections in which the researcher clarifies his or her particular perspective/s and relates this to the methods to be employed to collect, analyse and interpret data.

4.4 Research questions

Manson (1996:6) states that '. . . qualitative researchers should produce social explanations to intellectual puzzles'. The level of explanation inevitably depends on the question that is initially asked and the intention that the researcher has to theorise. Denzin and Lincoln (1998:8) leave open the debate regarding differing levels of interpretation and theorising when they write that qualitative researchers search for answers 'to questions that stress how social experience is created and given meaning'.

The research question in qualitative research is as important as it is in any other type of research. The question will help the researcher to choose an appropriate methodology, which in turn will enable the choice of data-collection methods. Phenomenologists pursue meaning of social phenomena via individual accounts of experience; ethnographers pursue understanding that is culturally constituted; and grounded theorists pursue explanations of social phenomena through inductively derived accounts of social situations. Action researchers do not necessarily address research questions. More typically they address a problem in practice.

Reflecting the complicated social world in which they practise, nurses reasonably ask questions that reflect that complexity. However, complicated questions have complicated answers. Qualitative research methodologies enable researchers to address complicated questions, but they rarely provide answers with positive formulas for practice. They provide propositional statements from which they and readers can infer reasonable responses that should improve service to people in similar circumstances to the study par-ticipants. For instance a study on the experience of receiving a blood transfusion (FitzGerald et al 1999) reports that in interview, adult inpatient respondents expressed differing degrees of worry regarding the likelihood, albeit small, of infection from a blood transfusion.

This information should cause nurses and doctors to reflect on their practice and plan to create better opportunities for patients to express doubts and receive individually appropriate support before and during blood transfusion. Note the recommendations are broad because the information does not lead to a prescription for all patients such as '. . . patients must have an information leaflet and sign a consent form that says they have received information'. The researchers in the blood transfusion study did not investigate the effectiveness of interventions to allay worry; they sought to understand the experience and revealed instances of worry despite there being a policy of informed consent for blood transfusion. The finding raises awareness of an issue; the reliance is upon readers to relate the information to their practice.

4.5 Methodology

Just four of the common methodologies used by nursing researchers are presented below. Bearing in mind that as these methodologies develop, they will continue to diversify, no particular approach deserves more attention than another in a chapter that gives such a broad overview. These examples should give the reader a taste of possibilities and the broad methodology that may suit their particular research interest and therefore are worth more thorough examination.

4.5.1 Phenomenology

Theorists such as Paterson and Zderad, and Dicklemann, Benner and Parse, introduced phenomenology as a research methodology in nursing. However, the most commonly used text to guide phenomenological researchers is written by an educationalist, Max van Manen (1990). In a vein similar to the other phenomenologists, Benner (Benner 1984, 1994) traces phenomenology through the work of the German philosophers, Husserl, Heidegger and Gadamer, and then to the influences from North America such as Dreyfus and Dreyfus. The importance of tracing the philosophical underpinnings of Benner's particular work should by now be obvious.

Phenomenologists use subjective experience of individuals to reveal a range of phenomena of interest to nursing. Everyday experience is collected as text using a range of data-collection methods (most commonly the unstructured interview). The data contain descriptions of social actions that are imbued with meaning. In an attempt to uncover raw experience, interviewees describe/portray their experience of a particular phenomenon with minimal direction in the form of questions. The researcher approaches the phenomenon with genuine curiosity and a belief that understanding lies in the everyday world. They do not follow hunches or prove points, and for this reason they do not usually review the literature before data collection. They critically reflect on their position and monitor and make explicit its effect on the emerging understandings. There are a number of methods for the analysis and interpretation of the phenomenological data. It is important to ensure that the method has congruence with the philosophical underpinning of the study, particularly in regard to the knotty phenomenological issue of whether or not to bracket—that is, to distance yourself from the interpretation (Walters 1994).

A typical pathway is one of immersion in the data and a hermeneutical interpretation that involves questioning of the text, fusion of horizons and movement from the parts to the whole of the text (Thompson 1990). This is a rigorous process at the same time as being a work of art in which the phenomenon of interest is portrayed as graphically as possible—indeed the reader of the phenomenological account should 'feel' the phenomenon.

Phenomenological research is useful for nursing in as much as it makes a humanistic contribution to disciplinary knowledge. Clients and nurses deserve to access accounts regarding the experience of particular interventions or circumstances, not to predict what might happen, but to be more aware. For example, anyone contemplating a course of chemotherapy should have access to information regarding the experience of others. A phenomenological account of this sort will enable the person to take stock of their situation, decide where they will be different and what they and their family might expect.

4.5.2 Ethnography

Madeline Leininger has led the way for nursing ethnographers. She used anthropology and ethnography as a means to develop her theory of nursing as a transcultural caring. However, Spradley is the early methodologist to whom reference is most commonly made when describing ethnographic methods of observation and key informant interviewing. He has written in detail about ethnographic interviewing and observation (Spradley 1980).

Ethnographers seek knowledge or understanding through the study of cultures—through cultural behaviours, cultural knowledge and cultural artefacts. Knowledge is assumed to be constituted by cultures; it is not thought to exist independent of any culture. This knowledge is attained through varying degrees of immersion in the culture and subsequent information gathering. The most common methods of data collection are observation (participant or non-participant), interviews of key informants (formal and informal) and reflective journalling.

The process of analysis and interpretation of textual data depends on the particular methodology used. Traditionalists will follow the reasonably prescriptive methods of 'developmental research sequence' described by Spradley (1980), while those with an interpretive perspective may use hermeneutic methods (Bull 2002), and critical ethnographers (Street 1995) will apply critique to the data and findings with an intent to change an aspect of the situation under study.

Some ethnographic studies provide important information about the way people from particular cultures experience our health services. Uncovering such meanings enables nurses to support these people to get what they need from the health service and have more opportunities for staying healthy. Information can also be learnt about the local culture in which we work and how rituals and symbols convey cultural meanings.

4.5.3 Grounded theory

Grounded theorists are interested in exploring social processes through human interactions (Streubert & Carpenter 1999). The methodology has been developed by Glaser and Strauss (1967) and later Strauss and Corbin (1998). It is informed by symbolic interactionism based on the premise that 'people behave and interact based on how they interpret or give meaning to specific symbols in their lives, such as style of dress or verbal and nonverbal expressions'

(Streubert & Carpenter 1999:103). Unlike more tentative methodologies there is intent by researchers using this methodology to build theory that is abstract, generalisable and testable.

Theory is built from empirical data; there is no attempt in grounded theory studies to apply a conceptual framework before data is collected. As with other inductive methods, a comprehensive literature review before data collection is not required because previous research findings may bias the collection of data and emergent theory. Streubert and Carpenter (1999:111) describe three steps:
1. reduction of data to codes and categories
2. use of the literature to relate to the concepts emerging from the data, and
3. selective sampling of data by collecting data specifically relating to the emerging ideas.

As data is collected it is analysed and compared with early results. This technique is called constant comparative analysis. As data is collected it is coded and through a process of comparison linked together to form categories and eventually an overriding theory. The amount of data collected is dependent on reaching 'saturation'—a rather nebulous term used to give scientific credibility to 'enough data'. Saturation is said to be achieved when recent data confirms the emerging theory and adds nothing new.

Grounded theory is well respected for its methodological rigour, and research students appreciate the methodical guidance that is less apparent in other qualitative methodologies. Results from grounded theory studies provide theory on a range of social phenomena to guide nursing practice.

4.5.4 Action research

In action research systematic change is used to generate knowledge through critical reflection on actions. It is underpinned by critical social theory that is explicitly political in nature and geared towards bringing about change in social situations. It is attractive to clinicians in its promise to engage and empower workers (clinicians) and to bridge the theory–practice gap. Pearson (1992) used action research in his study of the Nursing Development Unit at Burford. Hart and Bond (1995) and later Winter and Munn-Giddings (2001) have added much to action research in health service research. Winter and Munn-Giddings (2001) define action research as: 'the study of a social situation carried out by those involved in that situation in order to improve both their practice and the quality of their understanding'.

The research process is cyclical from an initial critique of the status quo that 'houses' the problem to planning, implementation, reflection and so on. Data collected to inform the researchers/participants in the research may be qualitative or quantitative. It is the critique of findings in situ and their immediate connection with the next cycle of action that makes action research so practical. This engagement with the situation by the researchers, and intention to influence that which is being studied, distinguishes action research from the other research methodologies, either qualitative or quantitative (Winter & Munn-Giddings 2001).

In theory, action research is ideological and attractive when first introduced to teams of clinicians. Many studies hit problems when busy clinicians cannot commit enough time to participation in the study. Winter and Munn-Giddings (2001:23) describe a 'culture of inquiry' necessary for successful action research—a culture where criticism is considered constructive and self-evaluation encouraged within a mutually supportive group. Such environments take time to build and maintain, and this is rarely taken into consideration when projects are first conceived.

Teams of practice developers use action research within their systematic and rigorous approach to person-centred care (Garbett & McCormack 2002). On a local level, action research is useful to nurses who want to be involved in research and to learn from their local situation. Published reports of action research can be useful templates for other teams who want to achieve similar changes in their service. The implementation of research evidence into practice and the evaluation of change is a current and constant imperative for all clinicians. Action research is a research methodology that has the potential to enable such implementation.

4.6 Evidence-based practice and qualitative findings

The contribution of qualitative findings to the whole EBP movement is explained in Chapter 5. How interpretive studies may be included in the systematic review and metasynthesis of propositional statements (findings) is relatively straightforward in theory. The process is much more difficult in practice when faced with multiple research studies pursuing the same phenomenon using a range of methodological nuances and apparently different language to represent the same thing (Thorne et al 2002, Sandelowski & Barroso 2002). Sandelowski and Barroso (2002) complain that it is sometimes difficult to identify the findings in reports of qualitative research. It is possible to synthesise the findings of qualitative research. The question is whether we would or should do so.

Meta-analysis and metasynthesis as the major techniques of EBP are by definition processes of reduction that run counter to most interpretive approaches. The notion that accumulated evidence for a particular position/finding renders the information more useful generally relies on the implicit belief of traditional science that 'more is better'. The verity of a qualitative study relies on the degree to which understandings arising from rich descriptions resonate as plausible to readers. Therefore it is reasonable to believe that a report that records three studies with the same findings does not ring truer than the single account.

However, there are schools of thought that believe that to exclude qualitative research from metasynthesis and the EBP movement is to deny its usefulness. The findings are enlightening and rely on the ability of the reader to translate them into different and better ways of practising. By synthesising the results and reporting them in a numerical way, they are at least being presented with authority to the world of practice. Involvement in the EBP movement does not necessarily detract from the stand-alone study and the impact that it may have on clinicians. From this perspective involvement in the EBP movement and creating metasynthesis of qualitative studies adds a string to the qualitative researcher's bow.

Examples of integrative reviews of qualitative research studies are relatively common nowadays. These combined studies have helped to draw attention to specific phenomenon and to guide new models of care that take into consideration subjective experience and the social world. Whether they do so with more authority than a single well-designed and reported study is still open to debate.

4.7 Critique

It is suggested that systematic reviews of the literature with explicit methods for appraising studies and extracting data has improved the quality of reporting of experimental studies. This may also be the case for qualitative research reports as Sandelowski and Barroso (2002:218), following a meta-analysis of qualitative research into the experience of women with Human Immuno-deficiency Virus (HIV) infection, report that there are problems with the quality of some research reports. They suggest that researchers need to 'find ways of reporting that accurately portray the lives they are meant to represent, but also to make findings discernible to the diverse audiences for whom they are intended, including researchers and practitioners'. Benner (1994) sums up the imperative for the interpretive researcher to balance the need to be creative and spontaneous with the need to produce an interpretation that is plausible, and which can be judged to be a 'good' or better' interpretation:

> *The method cannot transcend the talent or the moral character*
> *of the interpreter, but when the canons of textual evidence and*
> *consensual validation and dialogue are followed, a citizenry of*
> *critical readers and practitioners can discern better and worse*
> *interpretive accounts and better and worse ways of articulating*
> *common everyday taken-for-granted understandings. Practice then*
> *will have gained a way to influence and shape theory more directly*
> *and effectively (Benner 1994:124).*

Most research texts have a section regarding the critique of research reports. These frameworks are modified for qualitative research studies; however, they do not always take account of the particular methodology chosen by the researcher, and this type of clumping of studies under the one heading does not do justice to individual approaches. Classically qualitative research reports are long documents that include substantial methodology sections explaining and justifying the philosophical perspective and rich descriptions backed up by quotes taken from the raw data (all quotations should have a code that enables readers to relocate the words in their original context). The requirements of scientific journals for brevity and procedural writing are not conducive to 'good' reporting of qualitative research because so much information is necessarily left out.

4.8 Conclusion

This brief treatment of qualitative research has shown through an exploration of its generic characteristics that it does not stand in competition with quantitative research. Qualitative research addresses different research questions and uses different methodological approaches to do so. It represents an additional dimension of research that can be an excellent source of evidence for practice in nursing and other health services. Clinicians in all spheres of healthcare practice are exhorted to apply in their practice the evidence generated through research.

It has been cogently demonstrated in this chapter that evidence in this sense should not be construed narrowly and for nursing, in particular, the evidence generated through qualitative research cannot be ignored. As the nascent methodologies of qualitative research mature, they will become more prescribed and more refined in matters such as how results are reported. This may give more credibility to the evidence generated—but, already, the evidence abounds for the worth and value of enhanced understandings derived through qualitative research.

4.9 Discussion questions

1. Should the findings of similar qualitative studies be synthesised and summarised?
2. How are the findings of qualitative studies useful to clinicians?
3. Why would action research be the most appropriate research methodology for a team of clinicians who want to address a problem in practice?

4.10 References

Benner P 1984 *From novice to expert: excellence and power in clinical nursing practice.* Addison-Wesley, Menlo Park.

Benner P (ed) 1994 *Interpretive phenomenology: embodiment, caring, and ethics in health and illness.* Sage Publications, Thousand Oaks.

Bull R 2002 Theatre wear must be worn beyond this point, PhD thesis, University of New England, Armidale.

Denzin N, Lincoln Y 1998 *The landscape of qualitative research: theories and issues.* Sage Publications, Thousand Oaks.

FitzGerald M, Thorp D, Hodgkinson B 1999 Blood transfusion from the patients' perspective. *Journal of Clinical Nursing* 8(5):593–601.

Garbett R, McCormack B 2002 A concept analysis of practice development. *NT Research* 7(2):87–100.

Glaser B, Strauss A 1967 *The discovery of grounded theory: strategies for qualitative research.* Aldine, New York.

Hart E, Bond M 1995 *Action research for health and social care.* Open University Press, Buckingham.

Lincoln Y, Denzin N 1998 The fifth movement, chapter in N Denzin & Y Lincoln (eds) *The landscape of qualitative research theories and issues*, pp 407–29. Sage Publications, Thousand Oaks.

Manson J 1996 *Qualitative researching.* Sage Publications, London.

Pearson A 1992 *Nursing at Burford: a story of change.* Scutari Press, Peterborough.

Pearson A, Vaughan B, FitzGerald M 2004 *Nursing models for practice*, 3rd edn. Butterworth Heinemann, Oxford.

Sandelowski M, Barroso J 2002 Finding the findings in qualitative studies. *Journal of Nursing Scholarship* 34(3):213–19.

Spradley J 1980 *Participant observation.* Harcourt Brace, Fort Worth.

Strauss A, Corbin J 1998 *Grounded theory in practice.* Sage Publications, Thousand Oaks.

Street A 1995 *Nursing replay: researching nursing culture together.* Churchill Livingstone, Melbourne.

Streubert H, Carpenter D 1999 *Qualitative research in nursing: advancing the humanistic imperative*, 2nd edn. Lippincott, Philadelphia.

Thompson J 1990 Hermeneutic inquiry, in L Moody (ed) *Advancing nursing science through research*, pp 223–80. Sage Publications, Newbury Park.

Thorne S, Paterson B, Acorn S et al 2002 Chronic illness experience: insights from a metastudy. *Qualitative Health Research* 12(4):437–52.

van Manen M 1990 *Researching lived experience: human science for an action sensitive pedagogy.* SUNY, New York.

Walters A 1994 Phenomenology as a way of understanding in nursing. *Contemporary Nurse* 3(3):134–41.

Winter R, Munn-Giddings C 2001 *A handbook for action research in health and social care.* Routledge, London.

chapter 5

The systematic review process

Alan Pearson and John Field

5.1 Learning objectives

After reading this chapter, you should be able to:

1. *explain what is meant by a systematic review*
2. *construct an answerable question on which a systematic review could be conducted*
3. *conduct a systematic review, and*
4. *discuss the importance and effects of taking account of both quantitative and qualitative evidence.*

5.2 Introduction

The systematic review is critically important in the process of identifying the evidence on which to base practice. This is the tool that is used to locate the evidence and it involves the distillation from the literature of all of the evidence that exists for a given topic. In many respects, the systematic review is one of the great contributions to practice of the evidence-based practice (EBP) movement because it recognises that with the burgeoning healthcare literature—some two million new items each year—no practitioner can afford the time to keep abreast of it all, even if they had the ability. Systematic reviews have relieved practitioners to some extent of this burden because they bring together and assess all available evidence.

Before launching into a detailed consideration of the process of conducting a systematic review, it may help to clearly locate this step in the overall process of EBP. The steps involved in EBP are:

1. identification of an intervention, activity or phenomenon
2. determining the best available international evidence on this intervention, activity or phenomenon through a *rigorous process of systematic review*
3. development of recommendations for practice based on this evidence
4. development of practice guidelines based on this evidence together with local consensus

5. implementation of these guidelines, and
6. evaluation of the impact of these guidelines on the outcomes achieved by use of the intervention in accordance with the guidelines.

The systematic review (step 2) is a fundamental step in the process of EBP. It is, however, a detailed process that involves a significant commitment of time and other resources. This is particularly true if the review is to be exhaustive and there is little point to a review that is otherwise. Busy practitioners rarely manage to keep abreast of all of the current developments in their area of practice, much less have the opportunity to engage as individuals in the process of conducting a systematic review. Consequently, there are a large number of groups across the world that facilitate this process. There are a growing number of specialist collaborations, institutes and centres with skilled staff employed to train systematic reviewers, conduct systematic reviews and facilitate collaboration between reviewers.

5.3 The systematic review process

The systematic review is a form of research; indeed, it is frequently referred to as 'secondary research' (this is a reference to the source of data). Primary research involves the design and conduct of a study, including the collection of primary data from patients and clients and its analysis and interpretation. The systematic review also collects and analyses data—but usually from published and unpublished reports of completed research. Thus, the systematic reviewer uses a secondary source of data.

As in any research endeavour, the beginning point in the systematic review is the development of a proposal or protocol. After a subject is identified, protocol development begins with an initial search of two databases to establish whether or not a recent review report exists: the Cochrane Collaboration; and the Database of Abstracts of Effectiveness Reviews (DARE). If a review has been conducted it will almost certainly be found in one of these two databases. If the topic has not been the subject of a systematic review, a review protocol is developed.

5.3.1 Developing the review protocol

As in any research endeavour, the development of a rigorous research proposal or protocol is vital for a high-quality systematic review. The review protocol provides a predetermined plan to ensure scientific rigour and minimise potential bias. It also allows for periodic updating of the review if necessary. The following description of the development of a review protocol may seem overly prescriptive, but these are the steps that are required to ensure a high-quality review. Given that the consumers of the review are likely to be relying upon it for evidence upon which to base their practice, it is vital that reviews are of the highest possible quality. The development of a high-quality protocol requires the following:

- *Background review.* The initial step is to undertake a quick, general evaluation of the literature to determine the scope and quantity of the primary research, to search for any existing reviews and to identify issues of importance.
- *Objectives.* As with any research, it is important to have a clear question. The protocol should state in detail the questions or hypotheses that will

be pursued in the review. Questions should be specific regarding the patients, setting, interventions and outcomes to be investigated.

- *Inclusion criteria.* The protocol must describe the criteria that will be used to select the literature. The inclusion criteria should address the participants of the primary studies, the intervention or activity, and the outcomes. In addition to this, it should also specify what research methodologies will be considered for inclusion in the review (e.g. randomised controlled trials, clinical trials, case studies, interpretive studies).
- *Search strategy.* The protocol should provide a detailed strategy that will be used to identify all relevant literature within an agreed time frame. This should include databases and bibliographies that will be searched and the search terms that will be used.
- *Assessment criteria.* It is important to assess the quality of the research to minimise the risk of an inconclusive review resulting from excessive variation in the quality of the studies. The protocol must therefore describe how the validity of primary studies will be assessed and any exclusion criteria based on quality considerations.
- *Data extraction.* It is necessary to extract data from the primary research regarding the participants, the intervention, the outcome measures and the results. An effective way of systematically extracting data is to use a written protocol. An example of a protocol is shown in Figure 5.1. The protocol should be included as part of the report in order to afford transparency of method of extraction.
- *Data synthesis.* It is important to combine the literature in an appropriate manner when producing a report. Statistical analysis (meta-analysis) or textual analysis (metasynthesis) may or may not be used, and will depend on the nature and quality of studies included in the review. While it may not be possible to state exactly what analysis will be undertaken, the general approach should be included in the protocol.

The review protocol reproduced in Figure 5.1 is that used by the Joanna Briggs Institute (JBI).

5.3.2 Asking answerable questions

The assumption of EBP is that there are things we need to know in order to conduct our practice professionally. There are, however, substantial gaps in the knowledge available to us. Systematic reviews aim to expose the gaps in specific areas and provide pointers to the kinds of questions for which we need to find answers.

Sackett et al (1997:22) argue that almost every time a medical practitioner encounters a patient they will require new information about some aspect of their diagnosis, prognosis or management. This is no less true for other health professionals. They note that there will be times when the question will be self-evident or the information will be readily accessible. This is increasingly the case as sophisticated information technology gets nearer and nearer to the bedside. Even so, there will be many occasions when neither condition prevails and there will be a need to ask an answerable question and to locate the best available external evidence. This requires considerably more time and effort than most health professionals have at their disposal and the result is that most of our information needs go unmet.

Figure 5.1 The Joanna Briggs Institute review protocol

Title:

Background:

Objectives:

Criteria for considering studies for this review:

Types of participants:

Types of intervention:

Types of outcome measures:

Types of studies:

Search strategy for identification of studies:

Methods of the review:

Selecting studies for inclusion:

Assessment of quality:

Methods used to collect data from included studies:

Methods used to synthesise data:

Date review to commence:

Date review to complete:

Source: Reproduced with the permission of the Joanna Briggs Institute.

The first step is to have a question that is answerable. Asking answerable questions is not as easy as it sounds, but it is a skill that can be learned. Sackett et al (1997:30) offer some very useful advice in the context of evidence-based medicine and the effectiveness of interventions. These sources can be extended beyond questions of effectiveness, to consider the appropriateness and feasibility of practices. The source of a clinical question (adapted from Sackett et al 1997) is:

- *assessment*—how to properly gather and interpret findings from the history and physical examination and care
- *aetiology*—how to identify causes for problems

- *differential diagnosis*—when considering the possible causes of a patient's clinical problems, how to rank them by likelihood, seriousness and treatability
- *diagnostic tests*—how to select and interpret diagnostic tests to confirm or exclude a diagnosis, based on considering, for example, their precision, accuracy, acceptability, expense and safety
- *prognosis*—how to gauge the patient's likely clinical course and anticipate likely problems associated with the particular disease and social context of the person
- *therapy*—how to select therapies to offer patients that do more good than harm and that are worth the efforts and cost of using them
- *prevention*—how to reduce the chance of ill health by identifying and modifying risk factors, and how to detect early problems by screening and patient education
- *meaningfulness*—how to understand the experience of patients and the social context within which practice takes place
- *feasibility*—how practical it is to implement a practice within a given clinical setting, culture or country, and
- *self-improvement*—how to keep up-to-date, improve your clinical skills and run a better, more efficient clinical service.

Drawing on this, a clear, well-formulated question is developed to give focus to the systematic review. A clearly defined question should include specific details on:

- *The participants.* Participants should be defined clearly and this should include their condition (e.g. people with a confirmed diagnosis of emphysema), the population characteristics (e.g. females aged between 15 and 20 years), and the setting (e.g. in hospital medical wards).
- *The activities or interventions.* The question should specify the intervention or activity of interest (e.g. chest percussion or the administration of oxygen via a facemask).
- *The outcomes that are of interest.* The question should include the outcomes of interest to the review. The patient's satisfaction with care, peak flow or oxygen saturation levels are examples of the kinds of outcomes one might include in a review of interventions aimed at improving outcomes in people with emphysema.
- *The types of studies that are relevant to answering the question.* The question itself usually indicates the study designs that will be most appropriate. When the question focuses on experiences of people or communities, interpretive studies are usually indicated, whereas questions of feasibility may warrant economic evaluations and/or critical designs or evaluative designs. When the focus is on the effectiveness of a treatment, randomised controlled trials are considered to be the most appropriate, and questions relating to aetiology or risk factors may be best addressed by case-control and cohort studies.

Generally speaking, although health professionals often want to answer very broad questions, the narrower a question is, the easier it is to conduct the review. If the reviewers are interested in finding out the most effective, appropriate and feasible way of improving the quality of life for people with emphysema, it is desirable to conduct a series of reviews based on specific, focused questions rather than a broad, all-encompassing review that includes different populations, interventions and outcomes.

A well-formulated question will give direction to the search strategy to be pursued.

5.3.3 Finding the evidence

After you have identified the question, issue or problem from the field, the next step is finding the evidence. In order to do this it is necessary to have knowledge about the techniques used to unearth the evidence and make it available. Although systematic reviews and practice guidelines are designed to save practitioners time by presenting condensed information, it is important that these summaries of information are open to assessment. This can only be achieved by accessing the process used in the review. Just as research—published or unpublished—varies in quality, so can a literature search. Practitioners who want to base their practice on the best available knowledge need to learn new skills to access the resources available to help them.

5.3.3.1 The logistics of a search

In developing your search strategy, and then implementing that strategy, the logistics need to be well thought through. It is useful to be clear about:
- What databases/resources can be searched? Not all databases are accessible to reviewers and only those that can reasonably be utilised should be included.
- Who will do the search? Doing a comprehensive search is time-consuming, laborious and requires a degree of commitment. Someone who has the time, skill and commitment needs to be identified to do this, and a second reviewer with similar characteristics is also required.
- What help will be available from librarians? Although librarians may not be well versed in the substantive area of the review question, they are highly skilled in electronic searching and in the retrieval of papers. Conducting a search without the help of a librarian is not recommended.

The search strategy should be clearly described in the review protocol. Determining rigorous procedures for the search before commencing the review reduces the risks of error and bias. The first step in any search strategy is defining preliminary search terms or keywords, and then using these to search appropriate electronic databases. This preliminary search enables the reviewers to identify other keywords and to modify them according to the thesaurus used in each database. Databases most frequently used are:
- *CINAHL.* The Cumulative Index to Nursing and Allied Health (CINAHL) database provides authoritative coverage of the literature related to nursing and allied health. In total, more than 1200 journals are regularly indexed; online abstracts are available for more than 800 of these titles.
- *Medline.* Medline is widely recognised as the best source for bibliographic and abstract coverage of biomedical literature. It contains more than 9.5 million records from more than 3900 journals. Abstracts are included for about 67% of the records.
- *The Cochrane Library.*
- *PsycINFO.*
- *Current Contents.* This is an index of journal articles, reviews, meeting abstracts and editorials. It covers more than 7500 international journals of all disciplines, bibliographic information including English-language author abstracts for approximately 85% of articles, and reviews in the science editions.
- *DARE.*
- *AustRom.* This is a collection of Australian, New Zealand and Pacific region databases.

- *Science Citation Index.*
- *Embase.*
- *Dissertation Abstracts.*

See Chapter 1 for further discussion of some of these databases.

5.3.3.2 Conducting the search

Searching electronic databases is complex and requires a great deal of skill. It is important to work closely with a librarian in deciding which databases to search and what search terms to use in each of these. A number of potential problems can be avoided if a skilled librarian is involved. For example, differences in spelling conventions such as 'randomised' versus 'randomized' and 'paediatric' versus 'pediatric' can be overcome by using the thesaurus of specific databases and using various other techniques. The same applies when different terms are used in different countries (e.g. 'mucositis and 'stomatitis').

There are also variations in controlled vocabulary between databases. Medline, for example, uses the term Cerebrovascular Accident whereas in CINAHL the term Cerebral Vascular Accident is used to describe the same condition. Thus, when searching, it is important to utilise the aids available in databases. Truncation is an aid in some databases that can be used to search for a number of words with the same stem. In some databases, if an asterisk is inserted at the end of such a word (e.g. restrain*), then the search will include words that contain that stem (e.g. restraint, restrained, restraining).

Another useful aid is that of the 'wild-card'. A wild-card can be inserted in the place of a letter to pick up words that have different spellings. In some databases, the wild-card is used by inserting a question mark (e.g. randomi?ed) and any word with that spelling will be searched for (such as randomised and randomized). Most reputable databases have a thesaurus or controlled vocabulary, which is a list of headings used to standardise the indexing in the database. It is important to use this when conducting searches. It is also useful if you want to narrow or broaden your search to use an aid called Boolean operators. This aid is used by inserting the words 'and' or 'near' or 'not'. For example, if the term 'or' is used between terms, articles containing either term will be identified. So, if you searched for 'mucositis or stomatitis', you would get all the articles that had either mucositis or stomatitis in them. Searching for 'mucositis and stomatitis' would locate only those articles that contained both terms.

Not all journals are referenced in the electronic databases and many other sources of evidence, such as conference papers and unpublished work, will be lost to the review if it is limited to only electronic searches. A comprehensive review therefore also includes manual searching of journals and the reference lists of articles and abstracts retrieved.

5.3.4 Appraising the evidence

After you have conducted an exhaustive search, the resulting titles (and abstracts, if available) are assessed to establish whether they meet the eligibility criteria set out in the protocol. Those articles that do not meet the inclusion criteria are rejected but bibliographical details may be recorded in a table for inclusion in the systematic review report. Some reviewers do not include this in the report (e.g. Cochrane Reviews do not do so), whereas others do (e.g. Joanna Briggs Institute reviews include them as an appendix). If there is uncertainty about the degree to which an article meets the inclusion criteria, or if the criteria are clearly met, then the full text of the article is retrieved. Two reviewers then independently review all of the retrieved articles. If both reviewers agree to accept or reject an article, then the article is accordingly accepted or rejected. If there is disagreement between the reviewers on this issue, then the reviewers should confer and reach agreement.

Although published work looks impressive and authoritative, it is important for reviewers not to view it as unimpeachable or sacrosanct. That is to say, all work should be open to scrutiny and questioning. No work is perfect, but some is positively shoddy, and shoddy work must be weeded out. To a certain extent published work has been scrutinised if it is published in a peer-reviewed journal. However, it is most important that you are able to examine the work to identify what kind of evidence it has produced and how reliable or important that evidence is in terms of clinical practice.

Until 1999, evidence was ranked by quality in the National Health and Medical Research Council (NHMRC) (1995) *Guidelines for the development and implementation of clinical practice guidelines* in the following way:
- *I:* evidence obtained from a systematic review of all relevant randomised controlled trials
- *II:* evidence obtained from at least one properly designed randomised controlled trial
- *III–1:* evidence obtained from well-designed controlled trials without randomisation
- *III–2:* evidence obtained from well-designed cohort or case-control analytic studies preferably from more than one centre or research group
- *III–3:* evidence obtained from multiple time-series with or without the intervention (dramatic results in uncontrolled experiments, such as the results of the introduction of penicillin treatment in the 1940s, could also be regarded as this type of evidence), and
- *IV:* opinions of respected authorities, based on clinical experience, descriptive studies, or reports of expert committees.

However as detailed in Table 2.2 (see Ch 2), this was modified in 1999 (NHMRC 1999) to read:
- *I:* evidence obtained from a systematic review of all relevant randomised controlled trials
- *II:* evidence obtained from at least one properly designed randomised controlled trial
- *III–1:* evidence obtained from well-designed pseudo-randomised controlled trials (alternate allocation or some other method)
- *III–2:* evidence obtained from comparative studies with concurrent controls and allocation not randomised (cohort studies), case-control studies or interrupted time-series with a control group
- *III–3:* evidence obtained from comparative studies with historical control, two or more single arm studies or interrupted time-series without a parallel control group, and
- *IV:* evidence obtained from case series (either post-test or pretest and post-test).

This hierarchy of evidence was designed to assess the validity of recommendations for clinical guidelines and focuses, understandably, on the effectiveness of treatment. Phillips et al (1999) have developed, however, a broader frame to assess levels of evidence related to therapy/prevention, aetiology/harm, prognosis, diagnosis and economic analysis (see Table 5.1).

Table 5.1 Levels of evidence and grades of recommendations (23 November 1999)

Grade of recommendation	Level of evidence	Therapy/prevention, aetiology/harm	Prognosis	Diagnosis	Economic analysis
	1a	SR[1] (with homogeneity)[2] of RCTs[3]	SR (with homogeneity) of inception cohort studies; or a CPG[4] validated on a test set	SR (with homogeneity) of level 1 diagnostic studies; or a CPG validated on a test set	SR (with homogeneity) of level 1 economic studies
A	1b	Individual RCT (with narrow confidence interval)[5]	Individual inception cohort study with ≥80% follow-up	Independent blind comparison of an appropriate spectrum of consecutive patients, all of whom have undergone both the diagnostic test and the reference standard	Analysis comparing all (critically validated) alternative outcomes against appropriate cost measurement, and including a sensitivity analysis incorporating clinically sensible variations in important variables
	1c	All or none[6]	All or none case-series[7]	Absolute SpPins and SnNouts[8]	Clearly as good or better,[9] but cheaper. Clearly as bad or worse, but more expensive. Clearly better or worse at the same cost
	2a	SR (with homogeneity) of cohort studies	SR (with homogeneity) of either retrospective cohort studies or untreated control groups in RCTs	SR (with homogeneity) of level ≥2 diagnostic studies	SR (with homogeneity) of level ≥2 economic studies
B	2b	Individual cohort study (including low quality RCT; e.g. <80% follow-up)	Retrospective cohort study or follow-up of untreated control patients in an RCT; or CPG not validated in a test set	Any of: independent blind or objective comparison; or study performed in a set of non-consecutive patients, or confined to a narrow spectrum of study individuals (or both), all of whom have undergone both the	Analysis comparing a limited number of alternative outcomes against appropriate cost measurement, and including a sensitivity analysis incorporating clinically sensible variations in important variables

(continued)

Grade of recommendation	Level of evidence	Therapy/prevention, aetiology/harm	Prognosis	Diagnosis	Economic analysis
				diagnostic test and the reference standard; or a diagnostic CPG not validated in a test set	
	2c	'Outcomes' research	'Outcomes' research		
	3a	SR (with homogeneity) of case-control studies			
	3b	Individual case-control study		Independent blind comparison of an appropriate spectrum, but the reference standard was not applied to all study patients	Analysis without accurate cost measurement, but including a sensitivity analysis incorporating clinically sensible variations in important variables
C	4	Case-series (and poor quality cohort and case-control studies)[10]	Case-series (and poor quality prognostic cohort studies)[11]	Any of: reference standard was unobjective, unblinded or not; or independent; or positive and negative tests were verified using separate reference standards; or study was performed in an inappropriate spectrum of patients	Analysis with no sensitivity analysis
D	5	Expert opinion without explicit critical appraisal, or based on physiology, bench research or 'first principles'	Expert opinion without explicit critical appraisal, or based on physiology, bench research or 'first principles'	Expert opinion without explicit critical appraisal, or based on physiology, bench research or 'first principles'	Expert opinion without explicit critical appraisal, or based on economic theory

Notes:

1 Systematic review.

2 By homogeneity we mean a systematic review that is free of worrisome variations (heterogeneity) in the directions and degrees of results between individual studies. Not all systematic reviews with statistically significant heterogeneity need be worrisome, and not all worrisome heterogeneity need be statistically significant. Studies displaying worrisome heterogeneity should be tagged with a '–' at the end of their designated level.

3   Randomised controlled trials.

4   Clinical Prediction Guide.

5   Note that different considerations apply in understanding, rating and using trials or other studies with wide confidence intervals.

6   Met when *all* patients died before the Rx became available, but some now survive on it; or when some patients died before the Rx became available, but *none* now die on it.

7   Met when there are no reports of anyone with this condition ever avoiding (all) or suffering from (none) a particular outcome (such as death).

8   An 'Absolute SpPin' is a diagnostic finding whose <u>Sp</u>ecificity is so high that a <u>P</u>ositive result rules *in* the diagnosis. An 'Absolute SnNout' is a diagnostic finding whose <u>Sn</u>ensitivity is so high that a <u>N</u>egative result rules *out* the diagnosis.

9   Good, better, bad and worse refer to the comparisons between treatments in terms of their clinical risks and benefits.

10 By poor quality *cohort* study we mean one that failed to clearly define comparison groups and/or failed to measure exposures and outcomes in the same (preferably blinded) objective way in both exposed and non-exposed individuals, and/or failed to identify or appropriately control known confounders, and/or failed to carry out a sufficiently long and complete follow-up of patients. By poor quality *case-control* study we mean one that failed to clearly define comparison groups, and/or failed to measure exposures and outcomes in the same blinded, objective way in both cases and controls, and/or failed to identify or appropriately control known confounders.

11 By poor quality prognostic cohort study we mean one in which sampling was biased in favour of patients who already had the target outcome, or the measurement of outcomes was accomplished in <80% of study patients, or outcomes were determined in an unblinded, non-objective way, or there was no correction for confounding factors.

Source: *Available at www.cebm.net/levels_of_evidence.asp#top.*

This hierarchy of evidence takes a broader view of evidence but, like the NHMRC, renders all evidence that is not quantifiable as invalid for use in practice. Building on the Phillips et al framework, but taking a more inclusive view of evidence, Pearson (2002) reports on a hierarchy of evidence that includes the results of qualitative data (see Table 5.2).

5.3.5 The applicability of the evidence

There is little point in accumulating evidence to answer a question if we cannot then use that answer to benefit our patients. Remember, EBP involves the integration of best available evidence with your own clinical expertise. When it comes to deciding whether or not to incorporate into practice a particular activity or intervention, some or all of the following considerations will be relevant:

- Is it available?
- Is it affordable?
- Is it applicable in the setting?
- Would the patient/client be a willing participant in the implementation of the intervention?
- Were the patients in the study or studies that provided the evidence sufficiently similar to your own to justify the implementation of this particular intervention?
- What will be the potential benefits for the patient?
- What will be the potential harms for the patient?
- Does this intervention allow for the individual patient's values and preferences?

As well as needing to define levels of evidence for practice, there is also a need to establish levels of applicability. Pearson (2002) reports on the FAME scale (Feasibility, Appropriateness, Meaningfulness and Effectiveness) as a hierarchy of applicability of evidence (see Table 5.3).

Most systematic reviews are carried out by specialist centres and overseen by experienced systematic reviewers with substantial research experience. The systematic review process is also usually managed using software applications designed for the purpose. Spreadsheet software such as QuatroPro, Excel and Lotus, or database programs such as FoxPro or DataEase, are often used for electronic data collection and EndNote is increasingly used to manage bibliographical information. Review Manual (RevMan) and System for the Unified Management, Assessment and Review of Information (SUMARI) are programs designed to enable review teams to manage the systematic review process itself.

RevMan was developed by the Cochrane Collaboration. Users are able to enter a systematic review protocol, and then complete the review by entering information on each paper in the review including the characteristics of each paper, develop comparison tables, and enter study data. Of most use is the facility to conduct meta-analysis of the data, whether continuous or dichotomous, from quantitative studies. This facility also includes the ability to present the results of meta-analysis graphically in a format that is internationally recognised. RevMan is downloadable, at no cost, from the Cochrane Collaboration website and is used extensively across the world.

Table 5.2 Levels of evidence that include qualitative data results

Level of evidence	Feasibility F(1–4)	Appropriateness A(1–4)	Meaningfulness M(1–4)	Effectiveness E(1–4)	Economic evidence EE(1–4)
1	SR of research with unequivocal synthesised findings	SR of research with unequivocal synthesised findings	SR of research with unequivocal synthesised findings	SR (with homogeneity) of experimental studies (e.g. randomised controlled trial with concealed allocation) or one or more large experimental studies with narrow confidence intervals	SR (with homogeneity) of evaluations of important alternative interventions comparing all clinically relevant outcomes against appropriate cost measurement, and including a clinically sensible sensitivity analysis
2	SR of research with credible synthesised findings	SR of research with credible synthesised findings	SR of research with credible synthesised findings	Quasi-experimental studies (e.g. without randomisation)	Evaluation of important alternative interventions comparing all clinically relevant outcomes against appropriate cost measurement, and including a clinically sensible sensitivity analysis
3	SR of text/opinion with credible synthesised findings	SR of text/opinion with credible synthesised findings	SR of text/opinion with credible synthesised findings	3a Cohort studies (with control group) 3b Case-controlled 3c Observational studies without control groups	Evaluation of important alternative interventions comparing a limited number of outcomes against appropriate cost measurement, without a clinically sensible sensitivity analysis
4	Expert opinion without explicit critical appraisal	Expert opinion without explicit critical appraisal	Expert opinion without explicit critical appraisal	Expert opinion without explicit critical appraisal, or based on physiology, bench research or consensus	Expert opinion without explicit critical appraisal, or based on economic theory

Source: The Joanna Briggs Institute. Available at www.joannabriggs.edu.au/pubs/approach.php#B, viewed 8 August 2004.

Table 5.3 Levels of applicability of evidence

Grade of recommendation	Feasibility	Appropriateness	Meaningfulness	Effectiveness
A	Immediately practicable	Ethically acceptable and justifiable	Provides a strong rationale for practice change	Effectiveness established to a degree that merits application
B	Practicable with limited training and/or modest additional resources	Ethical acceptance is unclear	Provides a moderate rationale for practice change	Effectiveness established to a degree that suggests application
C	Practicable with significant additional training and/or resources	Conflicts to some extent with ethical principles	Provides limited rationale for practice change	Effectiveness established to a degree that warrants consideration of applying the findings
D	Practicable with extensive additional training and/or resources	Conflicts considerably with ethical principles	Provides minimal rationale for advocating change	Effectiveness established to a limited degree
E	Impracticable	Ethically unacceptable	There is no rationale to support practice change	Effectiveness not established

Source: The Joanna Briggs Institute. Available at www.joannabriggs.edu.au/pubs/approach.php#B, viewed 8 August 2004.

SUMARI is a developing program of the Joanna Briggs Institute (JBI). It is designed to assist reviewers to conduct systematic reviews of evidence of Feasibility, Appropriateness, Meaningfulness and Effectiveness, and to conduct economic evaluations of activities and interventions. The package consists of five modules:

1. *Module 1 Comprehensive Review Management System (CReMS)* is designed to accommodate the planning, monitoring and management of a systematic review. It includes the protocol, reviewer information, bibliographical information and time prompts. It incorporates the ability to import data from EndNote and includes fields to enter full data extraction and full critical appraisal documentation. CReMS has the capacity to generate publishing-house-standard systematic review reports and is suitable for researchers conducting systematic reviews that comply with the Cochrane Collaboration approach and for researchers who wish to incorporate other forms of evidence/data through the use of other SUMARI modules.

2. *Module 2 Qualitative Assessment and Review Instrument (QARI)* is designed to facilitate critical appraisal, data extraction and synthesis of the findings of qualitative studies.

3. *Module 3 Statistical Analysis Findings Assessment and Review Instrument (SAFARI)* is designed to conduct the meta-analysis of the results of comparable randomised controlled trials, cohort, time-series and descriptive studies using a number of statistical approaches.

4. *Module 4 Narrative, Opinion and Text Assessment and Review Instrument (NOTARI)* is designed to facilitate critical appraisal, data extraction and synthesis of expert opinion texts and of reports.
5. *Module 5 Analysis of Cost, Technology and Utilisation Assessment and Review Instrument (ACTUARI)* is designed to facilitate critical appraisal, data extraction and synthesis of economic data.

The CReMS module is web-based and, when downloaded on the user's server, can be accessed on the web by those authorised by the user. It can be used as a stand-alone program or in conjunction with other SUMARI modules.

Each of the other SUMARI modules are also web-based and are designed to interface with CReMS and all other modules.

The total package is designed so that each module interacts with the others and a reviewer can, at the point in the review when critical appraisal, data extraction and data synthesis/meta-analysis is reached, select a pathway to manage randomised controlled trials data, non-randomised controlled-trial quantitative data, qualitative data, textual data from opinion papers or reports, or economic data.

SUMARI is marketed commercially by the JBI.

5.4 Conclusion

The systematic review process is one element of the many steps involved in an EBP model. A knowledge of the systematic review process is not only vital for those who endeavour to partake in the process of conducting a systematic review but the understanding of the systematic review process is also of importance to healthcare professionals striving towards achieving EBP. This chapter has outlined the fundamental elements of the systematic review process and its importance to evidence-based information.

One of the strengths of a high-quality systematic review lies with the review question; a clear, well-defined research question will provide focus to the review. The steps to be undertaken in the review process should also be clearly described in the review protocol with particular reference given to the inclusion criteria and assessment of papers.

The appraisal of evidence is also an important aspect of the review process. Historically papers have been given rank according to the NHMRC levels of evidence. However, as highlighted, not all evidence is concerned with effectiveness and many well-designed papers go amiss when solely using this criterion. The SUMARI package provides the necessary tools to assist in the appraisal and synthesis of all forms of evidence from evidence of effectiveness to interpretive and critical papers, as well as papers founded in expert opinion.

Following the steps outlined in this chapter to conduct a systematic review will assist in achieving a high-quality review. It is important to remember when conducting a review that you are not alone; enlist the help of others, such as the librarian, and the systematic review process should be a smooth one.

5.5 Discussion questions

1. Systematic reviews of research involve the meta-analysis of data derived from primary research. Is secondary research a legitimate basis on which to ground practice?
2. What are the implications of including qualitative research in systematic reviews?
3. Given that systematic reviews are being advocated as a mechanism for evaluating evidence for practice, how can clinicians assess the quality of a systematic review?

5.6 References

National Health and Medical Research Council (NHMRC) 1995 *A guide to the development, implementation and evaluation of clinical practice guidelines.* Australian Government Publishing Service, Canberra.

National Health and Medical Research Council (NHMRC) 1999 *A guide to the development, implementation and evaluation of clinical practice guidelines*, 2nd edn. Australian Government Publishing Service, Canberra.

Pearson A 2002 Nursing takes the lead: redefining what counts as evidence in Australian healthcare. *Reflections on Nursing Leadership*, fourth quarter:18–21.

Phillips B, Ball C, Sackett D et al 2001 *Levels of evidence and grades of recommendations.* Centre for Evidence-Based Medicine, Oxford. Available at www.cebm.net/levels_of_evidence.asp#levels.

Sackett D L, Richardson W S, Rosenbery W, Haynes R B 1997 *Evidence-based medicine: how to practice and teach EBM.* Churchill Livingstone, New York.

part three

How to critically appraise the evidence

chapter ⑥ ─────────●

Effectiveness of nursing interventions

Anne Chang

6.1 Learning objectives

After reading this chapter, you should be able to:

1. *explain how a nursing intervention classification system has the potential to make the work of nurses more visible*
2. *distinguish among type I, II and III errors in determining the effectiveness of nursing interventions*
3. *identify methods for improving the strength of the nursing intervention in effectiveness studies*
4. *compare four methods of evaluating nursing intervention effectiveness in terms of differences between experimental and control groups, and*
5. *determine the types of evidence that can be used to judge the suitability of a nursing intervention for clinical use.*

6.2 Introduction

Determining the effectiveness of nursing interventions is essential for evidence-based nursing practice. Currently nursing practice is largely based on tradition and intuition with minimal consideration of the underlying scientific evidence, which leads to the further widening of the theory–practice gap (Estabrook et al 2003). Decisions in care are therefore often based on values and resources that are more opinion than evidence-based. However, the adoption of evidence-based practice (EBP) is likely to be influenced by the amount and level of evidence available, as well as the complexity of incorporating evidence into practice. This chapter will highlight factors related to the quality of the evidence of effectiveness of nursing interventions.

Since the initial recognition of the term 'nursing intervention' there has been extensive work on the further definition and elaboration. Nursing interventions are essential for the provision of health promotion and nursing care, and also provide a basis for the further development of nursing knowledge.

The large number and diversity of interventions necessitate a classification system to provide cohesion for the continued development and application. In appraising the quality of studies in systematic reviews of intervention effectiveness it is important to ensure that the intervention used is clearly described and administered with sufficient quality and strength. A strong and specific nursing intervention that is effective would have the capability to influence outcomes so that patients who received the intervention will differ from those who did not receive the intervention. Prior to translating the evidence into clinical practice, consideration of the feasibility, appropriateness and meaningfulness of the evidence for clinical practice and individual patients is essential.

6.3 What are nursing interventions?

Nursing interventions are undertaken for the benefit of clients with the nature of these defined by the scope of nursing. Nursing interventions arise from the identification of patient problems or nursing diagnoses, which identify the actual and potential health problems of individuals or groups (Snyder 1992, Carpenito 2000).

The first reported use of the term 'nursing intervention' found in the Medline database was in 1965. However, the more formal development of nursing interventions as essential components of nursing practice was not until the first two books published by Bulechek and McCloskey (1985) and Snyder (1985). These works contributed to the definition of nursing interventions and to the development of classification systems according to the major types of interventions.

The definition of the term 'intervention' within the remit of nursing has been of great benefit in delineating nursing practice. Such delineation will assist in making nursing more visible and identifying the contribution nurses make in healthcare through descriptions of the specific activities of nurses (Bulechek & McCloskey 1992). Examination of the different type or level of nursing intervention further assists understanding of the term. The level of independence of a nursing intervention is determined by the level of autonomy in decision making about the intervention (Snyder 1992).

Bulechek and McCloskey (1985) distinguish among the activities of the nurse on the basis of who initiates the intervention. When nurses use their knowledge base to make decisions on care, the interventions will be nurse-initiated or independent. Examples of independent nursing interventions include patient education, anxiety reduction and maintaining hydration. When other health professionals prescribe or order actions or therapies to be carried out by the nurse then the intervention is dependent, interdependent or physician (or other health professional) initiated. Interdependent nursing interventions denote those actions of the nurse that result from decisions made in collaboration with the healthcare team. Examples of this type of intervention include discharge planning and mobilising the patient. Dependent interventions are those actions that nurses carry out on the basis of other health professionals' prescriptions or orders. Examples include the administration of medications and the support and reinforcement of patient exercise regimens. Current work by the Iowa group on the classification of nursing interventions focuses on independent and collaborative interventions (see www.nursing.uiowa.edu/centers/cncce/nic/nicquestions.htm).

A nursing intervention classification system provides a more systematic organisation of the main activities of nursing, thereby facilitating research into therapeutic effectiveness and education (Snyder 1992). Furthermore such systems delineate the contribution of nursing in terms of quality of care and costs (Henry 1997). The development of these classification systems began in 1980 with the identification of the 10 main areas within the remit of nursing by the American Nurses Association (Snyder 1992). Seven types of nursing activities were identified in early work by Bulechek and McCloskey (1985). The Nursing Intervention Classification (NIC) is developed according to the seven domains of basic physiological, complex physiological, behavioural, safety, family, health system and community (see www.nursing.uiowa.edu/centers/cncce/nic/nicquestions.htm). Each intervention within the classification is defined and associated activities are outlined. From the initial development of 336 interventions there are now 514 interventions listed in NIC (Dochterman McCloskey & Bulechek 2004).

Other systems for classifying nursing interventions are the International Classification of Nursing Practice (ICNP) developed by the International Council of Nurses (ICN) (see www/icn.ch/icnpupdate.htm), the Omaha System for nursing interventions in community health (see http://cac.psu.edu/~dxm12/OJNI.html), and Home Health Care Classification (HHCC) (see www.dml.georgetown.edu/research/hhcc). Cross-mapping of the ICNP with the North American Nursing Diagnosis Association (NANDA) taxonomy I and NIC, Omaha System and the HHCC nursing intervention systems has been undertaken in an effort to develop a more unified and standardised language (Hyun 2002).

6.4 Effectiveness of nursing interventions

The delineation and classification of nursing interventions is crucial to the continued improvement in the quality of care and the ongoing development of nursing knowledge. Evidence-based care is founded in research on effectiveness of nursing interventions and is essential to ensure that the care provided by nurses is of benefit to patients. However, the testing of these interventions is often difficult with many methodological challenges in implementing the intervention. If a significant difference is found in an intervention study, checks are needed to assess whether or not a type I error has occurred (i.e. finding a difference when there is no real difference). Type I errors are more likely when the following design features are not present: random assignment to groups; double blinding; independence of groups; and level of significance (Schmelzer 2000).

All too often intervention studies have found no significant difference between the treatment and control or comparison groups (Closs & Cheater 1999). No significant difference may be due to a type II error, which means that the study was unable to detect the actual effectiveness of the intervention. The reasons for finding no nursing intervention effect are numerous and relate to study design matters such as: sample size and power of the study; selection of outcomes sensitive to the intervention; influence of extraneous factors; and timing of outcome measurement (Pruitt & Privette 2001, Schmelzer 2000, Clark 1996, Kirchhoff & Dille 1994). Many of these issues are addressed in texts on research methods.

Less frequently discussed is the validity and dose of the nursing intervention itself (Brooten & Naylor 1995). Descriptions of the usual care received by the control group are also important in evaluating the effectiveness of a nursing intervention. Effectiveness is more likely to be found where the intervention and the usual care are very different (Shuldham 1999). Sidani and Braden (1998) advocate that for research on effectiveness to have clinical relevance, greater attention is needed on the extraneous variables and the processes of the intervention, the use of representative clinical settings and a clearly developed theoretical basis for the intervention.

In effectiveness studies when conclusions are made that an intervention was ineffective when it had not been appropriately carried out represents a type III error (Sidani & Braden 1998). Such errors are unlikely in the more controlled laboratory setting and efficacy studies where the intervention is tested in the best possible circumstances (Muir Gray 2001). In an efficacy study of a nursing intervention a research nurse may be employed to provide the intervention (e.g. patient preoperative education) to all patients recruited to the experimental group. However, there are limitations in generalising findings from efficacy studies to the real clinical setting.

Research on effectiveness, in contrast to efficacy, is conducted in the clinical setting (Muir Gray 2001) with all the variability that entails and thus is more prone to type III error. There is difficulty in controlling the integrity and uniformity of the intervention in clinical effectiveness studies. Lindsay (2004) reports of findings of a systematic review of randomised controlled trials published from 2000 or 2001 in the *Journal of Advanced Nursing*. The author identifies the deficiencies in the reviewed papers as the absence of sufficient detail about the intervention or the usual care group. In the case of an effectiveness study of patient preoperative education, most of the nurses in the clinical setting would be delivering the education, thereby increasing variation in its implementation.

Strategies that have traditionally been used for reducing type III errors have included the development of an intervention protocol as well as training the interveners to follow this protocol (Polit & Hungler 1999). Pilot testing the protocol within the study setting will aid in developing a final protocol that accounts for the realities of clinical practice. Periodic checks on the adherence to the protocol can assist in ensuring the protocol is being delivered as designed.

More recent approaches to reducing type III errors include attention to the underlying theory of the intervention and process evaluation (Sidani & Braden 1998). The development of nursing-intervention classification systems can aid researchers in having clear and precise descriptions and understanding of the purpose of and actions comprising the intervention they are testing. Greater understanding of the strength or dose needed, whether the intervention has phases and which outcomes are appropriate for detecting an intervention effect will greatly improve the protocol developed for implementing the intervention. Furthermore this greater depth in understanding the intervention will enable the development of tools to undertake process evaluation.

6.5 How is the evidence validated?

Determining the quality of research on the effectiveness of nursing interventions requires the usual methodological checks as well as evaluation of the process of the intervention. Data on the strength, integrity, as well as timing and sustainability (Williams 2000) of the intervention, will assist in evaluating the degree to which the intervention was delivered as planned and the extent of subjects' participation (Flaskerud & Winslow 1998). The reason for process evaluation being infrequently reported in studies of effectiveness in nursing is likely to be due to the complexity of this evaluation.

Three different approaches to process evaluation include observation (Allen & Turner 1991), intervener self-rating scales (Egan et al 1992), nurse diaries (Forster & Young 1996) and patients' perceptions (Chang 1999). In a study of home-based psychosocial nursing interventions for myocardial infarction patients, Frasure-Smith et al (1997) reported the level of compliance with the protocol. However, it was unclear what compliance data had been collected, and it may have been more a measure of a patient's continuation in the research.

Furthermore the contextual factors such as the organisational setting may also have an impact on outcomes with an intervention producing certain outcomes in one setting but not in another setting. Brooten and Naylor (1995) indicate that nurse researchers are beginning to address the issue of generalisability of interventions across settings. They recommend continued effort in determining the dose of nursing intervention needed to achieve changes in patient outcomes.

6.6 Critical appraisal of quantitative evidence

The quality of the research can be determined by appraising the approaches to blinding, sample selection and randomisation.

6.6.1 Blind comparisons

The use of blinding to patient group allocation in clinical research enables control of bias that could arise from the study subject, the investigator, the data collector and/or data analyst knowing the treatment and placebo subject allocation, which could influence the response of the subjects and the outcomes measured (Portney & Watkins 2000, Schulz 2001). While double blinding is preferable it may not always be possible, such as for some types of clinical research (e.g. psychosocial nursing interventions or preoperative education where patients cannot be blinded to the intervention) (Shuldham 1999, Schulz 2001). Studies of effectiveness need to report the degree of blinding (i.e. whether the patients, researcher and/or data collector were unaware of patient allocation to groups).

6.6.2 Appropriateness of sample

The sample needs to be representative of the target population for the intervention study. It may be that the study sample is selected from an accessible population, as it would be difficult to contact all people in a target population. Whether target or accessible populations are identified, the sample needs to be representative, meeting the criteria for inclusion in the study. As indicated previously the greater the homogeneity of the sample the less the risk of committing a type II error.

6.6.3 Randomisation

The allocation of subjects to groups using a random process ensures that every subject has an equal chance of being allocated to a group (Polit & Hungler 1999). This process helps to avoid the bias that might arise with other methods of group allocation. Such misinterpretations of the effectiveness of interventions can be made when randomisation is not correctly applied.

Williamson (2003) in a systematic review of research articles published in the *Journal of Advanced Nursing* between 1996 and 2002 found that 68% used either convenience samples or the whole population, although many had reported using randomisation. It may be that randomisation is not possible given the interactive nature of a number of nursing interventions within a hospital or nursing-home setting. Patients randomly assigned to treatment and control groups may be in adjacent or nearby beds, which could result in contamination of the intervention. In such situations cluster randomisation would be preferable, so that groups or clusters of patients are assigned to the treatment and control groups (Polit & Hungler 1999).

6.7 Distinguishing between those who did and did not have the intervention

The aim in intervention studies is to determine if the outcome for those receiving the intervention differs significantly from those in the control group not receiving the intervention. These differences can be evaluated using four common methods (Altman 1994, Altman et al 2000): difference between means; risk difference; relative risks; and odds ratio.

6.7.1 Difference between means

Distinguishing among those who received and did not receive the intervention for scalar measurements is usually based on the difference between means, particularly if it is normally distributed. The outcome is the difference between the means of the two groups and the 95% confidence interval of that difference. The following provides an example:

> A controlled trial testing the effectiveness of two different types of wound dressing for leg ulcers had 105 subjects in the treatment group (dressing x) and 98 cases in the control group (dressing z). The mean healing rate for the treatment group is 1.58 cm^2/week $+/-1.5$ standard deviation (SD) and for the control group is 0.97 cm^2/week $+/-1.02$ (SD). The difference between groups $= 0.61$, the standard error (SE) of difference $= 0.18$, and the 95% confidence interval (CI) is 0.26 to 0.96. As this confidence interval has not overlapped zero (no difference), the null hypothesis can be rejected and the difference taken to be significant.

6.7.2 Risk difference

This approach is used for outcomes that are dichotomous where the risk is the percentage of the cases that has the outcome of interest or a positive outcome. This is commonly used to represent a change of risk following an intervention, such as occurred in a controlled trial. The result of the study is the difference between the risks of the two groups ($Risk_1 - Risk_2$) and the 95% confidence interval of that difference. The following provides an example:

In a controlled trial of washing hands before doing a surgical dressing, the treatment group (washing hands) has 150 cases, of which 20 had subsequent infections. The risk of this group ($Risk_1$) is therefore $20/150 = 0.13$. The control group has 120 cases, and 25 have infections. The risk of the control group ($Risk_2$) is $25/120 = 0.21$. The risk difference is $Risk_1 - Risk_2 = 0.13 - 0.21 = -0.08$, or an 8% reduction by washing hands. The 95% confidence interval is -0.19 to 0.04.

The conclusion is, therefore, that by washing one's hands one can achieve an 8% reduction in infections. However, as the confidence interval overlaps zero (no difference) this difference cannot be considered statistically significant.

6.7.3 Relative risks

This approach is similar to risk difference except that the ratio of the two groups and the 95% of that ratio is used instead of the difference in the risks. Although theoretically this should be used in epidemiological studies, by common usage it is also used in intervention studies.

Relative risk or risk ratio refers to the same statistical concept, to compare two risks by division, so that relative risk equals the risk in group 1 divided by the risk in group 2. That is, Relative risk = $Risk_1/Risk_2$.

In the same example as above, Relative risk = $Risk_1/Risk_2 = 0.13/0.21 = 0.62$. The 95% confidence interval is 0.37 to 1.09.

The conclusion is, therefore, that those washing their hands have 0.62 (62% or a bit more than half) the risk of infection than those not washing their hands. As the confidence interval overlaps the value of 1 (the same risk) this ratio cannot be considered statistically significant.

6.7.4 Odds ratio

The odds in a group refer to the number of cases with a positive outcome divided by the number of cases with a negative outcome. This can be demonstrated in the same example as above.

In group 1, 20 out of 150 developed infection, so that 130 (150 – 20) did not get infected. The odds of infection in group 1 are therefore $20/130 = 0.15$.

In group 2, 25 out of 120 developed infection, so that 95 (120 – 25) did not get infected. The odds of infection in group 2 are therefore $25/95 = 0.26$.

The outcome of a study is evaluated in terms of the ratio of the odds of one group divided by the odds of the other group and the 95% confidence interval of that ratio. This compares the odds of the two groups by division, so that the odds ratio equals the odds of group 1 divided by the odds of group 2. That is, Odds ratio = $Odd_1/Odd_2 = 0.15/0.26 = 0.58$, with a 95% confidence interval of 0.31 to 1.11.

Odds ratio was originally intended for use in case-control studies where risk could not be calculated, but common usage has also led to the use of odds ratio in intervention studies.

6.7.5 Evidence from meta-analyses

Although individual intervention studies do present evidence of effectiveness, the combination of similar studies (meta-analyses) is considered to present a higher level of evidence and inspire greater confidence in its conclusion.

Meta-analyses combine the results of an outcome of many studies and their 95% confidence intervals into a single outcome and its 95% confidence interval. The advantage of this type of analysis is that the combination of a number of studies increases the sample size so that if significant differences exist they are more likely to be demonstrated. That is, meta-analysis has the ability to increase the power of the evaluation of effectiveness of an intervention. Meta-analysis can be carried out using either difference between means, risk difference, relative risks or odds ratio; however, only one of these approaches is used in any single meta-analysis.

6.8 Is this nursing intervention suitable for clinical use?

As referred to in the chapter on outcomes (see Ch 8), evidence of effectiveness provides very important information for clinicians who want to be able to provide the best practice for their patients. However, an intervention may be found effective but considered to be impractical, inappropriate or meaningless to the patient, carer and/or health professional. Additional areas for consideration prior to implementing an intervention are the feasibility, appropriateness and meaningfulness of that intervention. The acronym of FAME has been adopted by the Joanna Briggs Institute (see www.joannabriggs.edu.au/related/sumari.php) to denote Feasibility, Appropriateness, Meaningfulness and Effectiveness.

6.8.1 Feasibility

The feasibility of an intervention relates to the practicality of applying this intervention in the clinical setting (see www.joannabriggs.edu.au/pdf/aboutQARI.pdf). While an intervention may have been found effective in the research setting it may not be feasible to use it in a less controlled setting where there may be a range of different levels of staff and the resources may restrict implementation. Research on the feasibility of particular interventions would aid health professionals in their decision making.

Gamel et al (2001) report a study involving the development of a sexual teaching nursing intervention for patients with gynaecological cancer, which was then tested for feasibility and acceptability. They used qualitative research methods to investigate the patient perspective on a pilot of the intervention, which found that the new intervention was feasible from the patients' perspective. The Feasibility Index developed by McDaniel (1999) provides elaboration of the meaning of feasibility of an intervention. This tool was designed to assess the feasibility of implementing a smoking cessation intervention for inpatients. The main elements in assessing the feasibility of implementing an intervention within the clinical setting were time, accessibility, coordination, receptivity, disturbance in the setting and communication with staff. McDaniel found the smoking cessation intervention had a high level of feasibility.

6.8.2 Appropriateness

Appropriateness can be seen in terms of the necessity for that intervention and also on the balance between benefits and risk of harm of an intervention. Appropriateness refers to the extent to which an intervention is suitable and fits with or is apt in a situation (see www.joannabriggs.edu.au/pdf/aboutQARI.pdf). Muir Gray (2001) identifies three categories of appropriateness of an intervention as those that are obviously appropriate or inappropriate and the third somewhere in between due to disagreements among clinicians and patients.

Qualitative methods may be more useful in determining the appropriateness of interventions. In a study of carers, appropriate interventions were those seen by Guberman et al (2003) to be focusing on care that carers believed was important, really needed and that may have been neglected. Gamel et al (2001:807) also recommend the use of qualitative studies to assist in developing an intervention that is appropriate or 'in harmony with the patient perspective'. The intervention, as indicated above in the section on feasibility, was for the purpose of sexual teaching for women with gynaecological cancer.

6.8.3 Meaningfulness

Meaningfulness of an intervention relates to the significance or importance the patient and family place on the intervention, thereby taking account of the particular circumstance of the patient (see www.joannabriggs.edu.au/pdf/aboutQARI.pdf)—that is, patients' appraisals or subjective interpretation of what is significant for them. Thus although there may be evidence of an intervention's effectiveness it may not be meaningful to the patient and family. The implications are that patient choice in the approach to care, and in this case, evidence-based care is required. However, while seeming to be desirable, integrating evidence with consideration of the meaningfulness is complex with little research available on such processes for deciding on care (Pearson 2004, Entwistle 1998). Meaningfulness is also seen to refer to the clinical significance of the evidence—that is, whether the evidence is important or significant in a particular clinical setting (Burns 2000).

6.9 Conclusion

Evidence of effectiveness of nursing interventions has the potential to guide nurses in adopting practices based on research evidence rather than on tradition and beliefs, and thereby to improve the quality of care provided. While EBP is preferred by many nurses today, the limited research on intervention effectiveness means that there often may be no available evidence. However, when evidence is available, caution is needed in critically appraising the quality of research to determine that the intervention and the testing of its effectiveness is valid. The adoption of practices reported in systematic reviews needs to be made in consideration of the thoroughness of the systematic review itself and the research under review. The articulation of nursing interventions and the associated classification systems provides a cohesive basis for use in research to test effectiveness.

A full and comprehensive definition of an intervention is an essential first step to testing and will increase the likelihood that the intervention is implemented with the strongest possible dose. Additionally the quality of the research can be determined by appraising the approaches to blinding, sample selection and randomisation. The methods for analysing the findings of the studies need to be able to clearly distinguish between the treatment and control groups. Prior to adoption of a particular EBP, attention is needed on the more qualitative elements of the intervention, namely the feasibility, appropriateness and meaningfulness of the intervention to patients and their families. Evidence is not for 'unthinking application', but for incorporation into the clinical decision-making process used in the provision of high-quality healthcare.

6.10 Discussion questions

1. A nursing intervention listed in the NIC system is 'swallowing therapy'. Define this intervention and list at least three associated, independent nursing activities for a patient with impaired swallowing.
2. Discuss how this intervention could be tested for effectiveness.
3. What might the patients' or carers' views be on the feasibility, appropriateness and meaningfulness of implementing swallowing therapy if it were found to be effective?
4. If the evidence of effectiveness is not of a high level (e.g. level 2 or 3 as in Table 6.1), should the intervention be adopted in the clinical setting?
5. Should current practice be changed on the basis of evidence from expert opinion?

Table 6.1 Levels of evidence of effectiveness

Level	Evidence of effectiveness
1	Systematic review (with homogeneity) of experimental studies (e.g. randomised controlled trial with concealed allocation), or one or more large experimental studies with narrow confidence intervals
2	Quasi-experimental studies (e.g. without randomisation)
3a	Cohort studies (with control group)
3b	Case-controlled
3c	Observational studies without control groups
4	Expert opinion without explicit critical appraisal, or based on physiology, bench research or consensus

Source: The Joanna Briggs Institute. Available at www.joannabriggs.edu.au/pubs/approach.php.

6.11 References

Allen C I, Turner P S 1991 The effect of an intervention programme on interactions on a continuing care ward for older people. *Journal of Advanced Nursing* 16(10):1172–7.

Altman D G 1994 *Practical statistics for medical research*, 2nd edn, pp 233–68. Chapman Hall, London.

Altman D G, Machin D, Bryant T N, Gardner M J 2000 *Statistics with confidence*, 2nd edn, pp 57–67 and 121–2. BMJ Books, London.

Brooten D, Naylor M D 1995 Nurses' effect on changing patient outcomes. *Image: The Journal of Nursing Scholarship* 27(2):95–9.

Bulechek G M, McCloskey J V (eds) 1985 *Nursing interventions: treatments for nursing diagnoses*. WB Saunders, Philadelphia.

Bulechek G M, McCloskey J V 1992 *Nursing interventions: essential nursing treatments*, 2nd edn. WB Saunders, Philadelphia.

Burns K J 2000 Power and effect size: research considerations for the clinical nurse specialist. *Clinical Nurse Specialist* 14(2):61–8.

Carpenito L J 2000 *Nursing diagnosis: application to clinical practice,* 8th edn. Lippincott, Philadelphia.

Chang A M 1999 Psychosocial nursing intervention to promote self-esteem and functional independence following stroke. Unpublished PhD dissertation, the Chinese University of Hong Kong.

Clark A J 1996 Optimizing the intervention in research studies. *Advanced Practice Nursing Quarterly* 2(3):1–4.

Closs S J, Cheater F M 1999 Evidence for nursing practice: a clarification of the issues. *Journal of Advanced Nursing* 30(1):10–17.

Dochterman McCloskey J, Bulechek G M 2004 *Nursing interventions classification (NIC)*, 4th edn. Mosby, St Louis.

Egan E C, Snyder M, Burns K R 1992 Intervention studies in nursing: is the effect due to the independent variable? *Nursing Outlook* 40(4):187–90.

Entwistle V A, Sheldon T A, Sowden A, Watt I S 1998 Evidence-informed patient choice. Practical issues of involving patients in decisions about health care technologies. *International Journal of Technology Assessment in Health Care* 14(2):212–25.

Estabrook C A, Floyd J A, Scott-Findlay S et al 2003 Individual determinants of research utilization: a systematic review. *Journal of Advanced Nursing* 43(5):506–20.

Flaskerud J H, Halloran E J, Janken J et al 1979 Avoiding and distancing a descriptive view of nursing. *Nursing Forum* 18(2):158–74.

Flaskerud J H, Winslow B J 1998 Conceptualizing vulnerable populations' health-related research. *Nursing Research* 47(2):69–78.

Forster A, Young J 1996 Specialist nurse support for patients with stroke in the community: a randomised controlled trial. *British Medical Journal* 312(7047):1642–6.

Frasure-Smith N, Lesperance F, Prince R H et al 1997 Randomised trial of home-based psychosocial nursing intervention for patients recovering from myocardial infarction. *The Lancet* 350(9076):473–9.

Gamel C, Grypdonck M, Hengeveld M, Davis B 2001 A method to develop a nursing intervention: the contribution of qualitative studies to the process. *Journal of Advanced Nursing* 33(6):806–19.

Gould D, James T, Tarpey A et al 2000. Intervention studies to reduce the prevalence and incidence of pressure sores: a literature review. *Journal of Clinical Nursing* 9(2):163.

Guberman N, Nicholas E, Nolan M et al 2003 Impacts on practitioners of using research-based carer assessment tools: experiences from the UK, Canada and Sweden, with insights from Australia. *Health and Social Care in the Community* 11(4):345–55.

Henry S B 1997 Comparison of Nursing Interventions Classification and Current Procedural Terminology codes for categorizing nursing activities. *Image: Journal of Nursing Scholarship* 29(2):133–8.

Home Health Care Classification (HHCC). Available at www.dml.georgetown.edu/research/hhcc.

Hyun S 2002 Cross-mapping the ICNP with NANDA, HHCC, Omaha system and NIC for unified nursing language system development. *International Nursing Review* 49(2):99–110.

International Council of Nurses (ICN). Available at www/icn.ch/icnpupdate.htm.

Joanna Briggs Institute (JBI). Available at www.joannabriggs.edu.au/related/sumari.php.

Kirchhoff K T, Dille C A 1994 Issues in intervention research: maintaining integrity. *Applied Nursing Research* 7(1):32–46.

Lindsay B 2004 Randomized controlled trials of socially complex nursing interventions: creating bias and unreliability? *Journal of Advanced Nursing* 45(1):84–94.

McDaniel A M 1999 Assessing the feasibility of a clinical practice guideline for inpatient smoking cessation intervention. *Clinical Nurse Specialist* 13(5):228–35.

Muir Gray J A 2001 Evidence-based healthcare. How to make health policy and management decisions, 2nd edn. Churchill Livingstone, New York.

Nursing Intervention Classification (NIC). Available at www.nursing.uiowa.edu/centers/cncce/nic/nicquestions.htm.

Omaha System. Available at http://cac.psu.edu/~dxm12/OJNI.html.

Pearson A 2004 Balancing the evidence: incorporating the synthesis of qualitative data into systematic reviews. *JBI Reports* 2(2):45–64.

Polit D F, Hungler B P 1999 *Nursing research: principles and methods*, 2nd edn. Lippincott, Philadelphia.

Portney L G, Watkins M P 2000 *Foundations of clinical research: applications to practice*, 2nd edn. Prentice Hall Health, Upper Saddle River.

Pruitt R H, Privette A 2001 Planning strategies for the avoidance of pitfalls in intervention research. *Journal of Advanced Nursing* 35(4):514–20.

Schmelzer M 2000 Understanding the research methodology: should we trust the researchers' conclusions? *Gastroenterology Nursing* 23(6):269–74.

Shuldham C 1999 Pre-operative education: a review of the research design. *International Journal of Nursing Studies* 36(2):179–87.

Schulz K F 2001 Assessing allocation concealment and blinding in randomised controlled trials: why bother? (editorial). *Evidence-based Nursing* 4(1):4–6.

Sidani S, Braden C J 1998 *Evaluating nursing interventions: a theory-driven approach*. Sage Publications, Thousand Oaks.

Snyder M 1985 *Independent nursing interventions*. John Wiley, New York.

Snyder M 1992 *Independent nursing interventions*, 2nd edn. Delmar, Albany, New York.

Williams L A 2000 Creating sustainable nursing interventions: an innovative health promotion strategy for handwashing in child care centres. *Neonatal Paediatric Child Health Nursing* 3(4):17–20.

Williamson G R 2003 Misrepresenting random sampling? A systematic review of research papers in the *Journal of Advanced Nursing*. *Journal of Advanced Nursing* 44(3):278–88.

chapter (7)

Assessing the effectiveness of screening and diagnostic tests

Wendy Chaboyer and Lukman Thalib

7.1 Learning objectives

After reading this chapter, you should be able to:

1. *understand what screening and diagnostic tests are and why they are used*
2. *identify commonly used screening and diagnostic tests in health*
3. *critically appraise the sensitivity, specificity, likelihood ratio and receiver operator characteristic curve of screening and diagnostic tests, and*
4. *assess the usefulness of screening and diagnostic tests.*

7.2 Introduction

As part of everyday clinical practice nurses assess patients and make judgments about their real or potential health problems. Based on these judgments nurses will initiate a variety of interventions. At times, formal tests or other investigatory instruments are used to aid in this judgment. When tests are used, it is important that they are able to correctly distinguish between those with and without the particular problem. Two types of tests, screening and diagnostic, are described in this chapter. After providing an overview of the tests, including why they may be undertaken, issues of test accuracy are addressed. Next, guidelines for critical appraisal of screening and diagnostic tests are outlined. Finally, the chapter describes issues to be considered when making decisions about the use of screening and diagnostic tests.

7.3 What are screening and diagnostic tests?

Screening, or mass health screening as it is often known, involves the use of a test or other investigatory instrument to detect individuals at risk of developing some specific disease or health condition that is amenable to effective prevention or treatment. In other words, screening is a population-based strategy to identify specific conditions in people who have not sought medical care for any concerns related to that disorder in question (Kerr et al 1998). Screening tests can be used on the whole population, such as the phenylketonuria (PKU) test done on all newborns, or they can be used on sub-groups, such as mammograms for women who have a family history of breast cancer. There are many common screening tests used in nursing. Falls risk assessment tools (Eagle et al 1999, Mercer 1997, Perell 2001) and pressure ulcer risk assessment tools (Anthony et al 2000, Woodbury et al 1999) are two examples clinical nurses may be familiar with.

While screening tests seek to identify those at risk, diagnostic tests are measures used to identify individuals who actually have health problems or conditions and who will benefit from treatment (Newman et al 2001). It should be clear that screening tests are not diagnostic tests and diagnosis is in fact the next sequence in the screening pathway to confirm or reject an abnormality identified by the screening test. While doctors use a vast majority of diagnostic tests, they are used less frequently in nursing. One example of diagnostic tests used by nurses is the sedation scales (Ramsey et al 1974, Marx et al 1994, Young-McCaughan & Miaskowski 2001).

For diagnostic tests to be useful, there must be some beneficial treatment that results from detecting the problem or condition. The basic underlying assumption for both screening and diagnostic tests is that early detection will lead to better care and ultimately better outcomes. While screening and diagnostic tests are used for two different purposes, the first of which is to detect those at risk for some condition and the second to actually detect a specific condition, consideration of utility, accuracy and feasibility of both is similar. This chapter presents principles that can be applied to make judgments about both screening and diagnostic tests.

7.4 Why are screening and diagnostic tests undertaken?

Screening and diagnostic tests are used to identify individuals who do not have signs or symptoms of some problem or condition, but who would benefit from early identification, diagnosis and treatment. Several basic principles should be considered when deciding whether to begin a screening program (Hennekens & Buring 1987). First, the problem or condition that the test is meant to detect must be serious enough to warrant testing. Second, it should be either fairly common or, if rare, have serious effects. Third, it must be amenable to some form of treatment that will be beneficial. Fourth, there must be adequate resources to manage the follow-up care and treatment. Fifth, the follow-up care and treatment should be acceptable to the individuals receiving it. Finally, the test should be accurate.

Two examples of screening tests include blood pressure monitoring for hypertension and risk assessment screening for falls in the elderly. Hypertension, often known as the silent killer, is a serious and a common condition that is thought to affect up to one-quarter of the population and carries with it a risk of death. Both the screen (blood pressure monitoring) and the treatment are acceptable to the community. Additionally, treatment has been shown to reduce morbidity and mortality considerably.

104

Another well-known example for nurses is falls in the elderly, which occur less frequently. However, when they do occur they have the potential to have devastating effects (Cutson 1994). There are several strategies that can be implemented to diminish the likelihood of falling. However, if there are not enough resources to initiate some additional care or treatment for those identified as at risk of falling, then the use of the assessment tool has little benefit. Similarly, the additional care an individual receives as a result of being at risk of falling must be acceptable to the person. Finally, if the risk assessment does not identify those who are really at risk or identifies a lot of individuals who are not at risk of falling, then many people will get unnecessary care and treatment, while others who need monitoring may not receive it. This notion of test accuracy is a very important consideration and is dealt with in more detail in the next section.

7.5 Is the screening or diagnostic test accurate?

When considering whether a test is accurate, a clinician must understand how the test was assessed for accuracy. The basic research question that is answered in studies on test accuracy is 'to what extent does the test give the right answer?' (Newman et al 2001:179). While it may appear self-evident that accuracy is important, a significant proportion of studies do not report this information. For example, in the review on patient falls conducted by Perell et al (2001), only eight out of 15 articles on risk-assessment tools provided this information. Evaluation of a test requires both the use of a valid research design to collect information on the test and appropriate statistical analyses of the data that is collected. Issues related to study design of screening tests and diagnostic tests are given below, followed by statistical measures that are used to quantify the characteristics of tests.

7.5.1 Screening tests

Researchers generally use randomised controlled trials or cohort studies to test the accuracy of screening tests (Muir Gray 1997). In randomised controlled trials, individuals are randomly allocated to one of two groups (screening or no screening), and then some outcome such as mortality or morbidity is assessed (Newman et al 2001). It is important that these outcomes are identified because researchers want to establish that undertaking the screening has benefits beyond simply early diagnosis. That is, if early diagnosis does not lead to better outcomes, then the screening test is not worthwhile. It is important to remember that, due to a variety of methodological and ethical issues, not all screening tests are amenable to randomised controlled trial assessment; however, randomised controlled trials are the best design to determine test accuracy.

In cohort studies assessing the accuracy of a screening test, the morbidity or mortality of those screened is compared to those who choose not to be screened (Newman et al 2001). Difficulties associated with using a cohort study include self-selection bias and lead-time bias. Self-selection bias is the term used to describe the fact that individuals who decide to get tested may be different in some way to those who choose not to get tested (Hennekens & Buring 1987). Lead-time bias is defined as the interval between diagnosis of some problem or condition at screening and when it would have been identified due to the development of symptoms (Hennekens & Buring 1987). Lead-time will vary according to the problem or condition that is being screened. However, if it is not taken into consideration, then screening may appear to be more beneficial than it really is.

An example may assist in understanding the importance of lead-time bias. Two people develop hypertension at the age of 40. The first is diagnosed after screening at age 52 and the second is diagnosed because of headache and dizziness at age 62; however, both die of a massive stroke at age 72. The first person lived 20 years and the second lived 10 years after diagnosis, and so it appears that the screening was effective; however, they still both developed the condition and died at the same age. The only thing the screening did was detect the problem earlier.

7.5.2 Diagnostic tests

In studies to assess the accuracy of diagnostic tests, correlational research is often used to compare the results of the diagnostic test to the results obtained from some reference standard (Newman et al 2001), often termed the 'gold standard'. The results of the diagnostic test should be similar to that of the reference standard, in terms of those who do and do not have the problem or condition. Importantly, all individuals in the study should receive both the diagnostic test and the reference standard, and those who are interpreting the test should be blinded to the results of the standard and vice versa (Begg 1987).

While this seems relatively clear, consider the use of ventilation-perfusion scans to identify pulmonary embolism. If individuals get a negative scan result, clinicians may be hesitant to subject them to the more invasive gold standard test, angiography. Thus, some individuals may receive the diagnostic test but do not receive the gold standard, a phenomenon termed verification bias (Begg 1987). There is also the potential for bias to develop if the two tests were not performed independently. That is, if the results of one test are known when the second test is being assessed, then bias may be introduced. Additionally, while a diagnostic test may be able to identify those at the severe end of the spectrum, if it is not able to identify those with milder forms of the problem or condition, then spectrum bias may be an issue (Fischer et al 2003). This means that the sample should contain a wide variation in the spectrum of the problem or condition, from mild to severe.

7.6 Does the test identify those with the problem?

This section will acquaint you with the basics of assessing the value of screening and diagnostic tests. The most common use of the knowledge of assessment of a test comes when a patient has an abnormal pathology result and you wonder 'What does this really mean?' and 'How likely is it that this patient really has the problem or condition in question?' For example, take a case of a 50-year-old woman who had a routine mammogram that is interpreted as 'positive'. What is the probability of this woman with a positive mammogram actually having breast cancer? This is a practical question that nurses and other clinicians face every day. Understanding some of the basic concepts of test interpretation will help you make better decisions about test ordering and interpretation.

7.6.1 Sensitivity, specificity and predictive values

Although screening tests are meant to identify those who are at risk of developing a health problem or condition and diagnostic tests are meant to identify those with the problem or condition prior to any signs or symptoms arising, few tests are perfect. A good test will correctly identify those that truly are at risk of, or actively having, the problem or condition, termed *true positives*. Likewise it will correctly identify those who are not at risk or do not have the problem or condition, termed *true negatives*. Sometimes the test will incorrectly classify some people as being at risk of or actually having the problem or condition when they do not, termed *false positives*. Likewise, it can incorrectly classify them as not being at risk of or having the problem or condition, when in fact they do, termed *false negatives*. Thus, when a test is administered, there are four possible results: true positive; true negative; false positive; and false negative.

Sensitivity and specificity are the terms used to describe the relationship between true and false positives and negatives. The sensitivity of a test is the proportion of people with the problem or condition who are detected as having it when the test is used (true positives). The specificity of a test is the proportion of people without the problem or condition who are detected as not having it when the test is used (true negatives).

Figure 7.1 displays the relationship between the problem or condition in reality and the test results. Mathematically, sensitivity can be calculated using the following formula:

$$\text{Sensitivity} = \frac{\text{True positives}}{\text{True positives} + \text{False negatives}}$$

Alternatively using the symbols given in Figure 7.1:

$$\text{Sensitivity} = \frac{a}{a + c}$$

Likewise:

$$\text{Specificity} = \frac{\text{True negatives}}{\text{True negatives} + \text{False positives}}$$

Or using the symbols in Figure 7.1:

$$\text{Specificity} = \frac{d}{b + d}$$

Sensitivity and specificity describe how well the test discriminates between the population of patients with and without the disease. They address a different question than we want answered when evaluating an individual patient. What we usually want to know is, given a certain result, what is the probability of a disease? This leads to the concept of predictive values (PVs). 'Predictive values measure whether or not an individual actually has the disease, given the result of the screening test' (Hennekens & Buring 1987:336). PVs help to determine the number of cases that will be detected by a screening program, sometimes termed yield. A positive PV is the probability of a problem when the test is positive and is denoted as $PV+ = \dfrac{a}{a+b}$ when referring to Figure 7.1 (Dujardin et al 1994). A negative PV is the probability of the absence of a problem if the test is negative and is denoted as $PV- = \dfrac{d}{c+d}$ when referring to Figure 7.1. The formulas for PV demonstrate that they are influenced by the prevalence of the problem in the population. That is, an increase in prevalence will increase the positive PV of a test, which is one reason why PVs can be limited in value (Dujardin et al 1994).

The results from a test are not always dichotomous (i.e. positive or negative), but rather can sometimes be continuous, or have a large number of response options. Take, for example, the results of a blood-sugar level. They can range from under three to over 20 mmol/l. At what point do we decide that the individual is hyperglycaemic? Some cut-off point must be established and when this cut-off point is exceeded, then an individual is said to be hyperglycaemic. Altering this criterion of positive test result will influence both the sensitivity and specificity of the test (Hennekens & Buring 1987). Making a cut-off for a positive test result less stringent will result in more individuals who actually have the problem or condition testing positive (increased sensitivity), but it will also increase the number testing positive that do not have it (decreased specificity). Likewise, making the criterion more stringent will mean that more individuals who test negative will actually not have the problem or condition (increased specificity), but more individuals with the problem or condition will be missed (decreased sensitivity). The next section provides more information on this topic by describing likelihood ratios, a method for describing test accuracy when the test uses a continuous measure.

Figure 7.1 Potential test results

Test results		Reference or gold standard		
		Present	Absent	
Test results	Positive	True positive (a)	False positive (b)	Predictive value + = a/(a + b)
	Negative	False negative (c)	True negative (d)	Predictive value − = d/(c + d)
		Sensitivity = a/(a + c)	Specificity = d/(b + d)	
		$LR+ = \dfrac{\text{Sensitivity}}{(1 - \text{Specificity})}$	$LR- = \dfrac{(1 - \text{Sensitivity})}{\text{Specificity}}$	

7.6.2 Likelihood ratios

Likelihood ratios (LRs) are an alternative method of assessing the performance of a diagnostic test. The main advantage of LRs is that they can deal with tests with more than two possible results. An LR is the ratio of the likelihood of the results in someone with the problem or condition to the likelihood of that same result in someone who does not have it (Fischer et al 2003). In essence, an LR summarises the sensitivity and specificity information of a test. If the test is dichotomous then the likelihood ratio for a positive test is $LR+ = \dfrac{\text{Sensitivity}}{1 - \text{Specificity}}$ and the LR for a negative test is $LR- = \dfrac{1 - \text{Sensitivity}}{\text{Specificity}}$. The higher the LR (greater than 1), the better the test is for ruling in a problem or condition, while the lower the likelihood ratio (closer to 0), the better the test is for ruling out a problem or condition (Newman et al 2001). An LR of 1 provides no information about the likelihood of a problem or condition (Newman et al 2001), and suggests that the test is of no value (Dujardin et al 1994). The following case study provides a working example of the concepts of sensitivity, specificity, predictive values and likelihood ratios. It demonstrates how these concepts are calculated and the relationship among them. In this example, iron deficiency anaemia has been confirmed using a gold standard and serum ferritin is the diagnostic test used. Refer to Figure 7.2 when reading the case study.

Case study: Calculations for measures quantify the characteristics of a test

The serum ferritin level was tested in a population of 750 individuals (250 + 50 + 25 + 425), 300 of whom were confirmed to have an iron deficiency anaemia (250 + 50). The other 450 individuals were confirmed to *not* have iron deficiency anaemia (25 + 425). However, the serum ferritin test identified that 275 individuals had iron deficiency anaemia (250 + 25). So there is a discrepancy between the confirmed cases of 300 and the diagnostic test cases of 275. There is also a discrepancy between the number identified by serum ferritin—that is, 475 (50 + 425)—as compared to those 450 confirmed to not have iron deficiency anaemia.

Using the formulas provided, serum ferritin (the diagnostic test) has a sensitivity of 83%, which means that 83% of those who have anaemia in this particular population were correctly identified by the diagnostic test. It has a specificity of 94%, which means that 94% of those who do not have anaemia in this particular population were correctly identified as negative by the test.

The calculated positive predictive value of 91% means that when an individual tests positive on the serum ferritin test he or she has a 91% chance of actually having iron deficiency anaemia. And, when an individual

---

tests negatively, the negative predictive value identifies that he or she has an 89% chance of *not* having iron deficiency anaemia.

We can compare the probability of getting any test result if the patient truly had the iron deficiency anaemia versus if the patient was healthy using likelihood ratios. The calculated positive likelihood ratio of 13.8 demonstrates that a positive serum ferritin test identifying the patient actually having iron deficiency anaemia is 14 times more than wrongly diagnosing someone who has no anaemia. Any positive likelihood ratio of over 10 is generally considered large and often indicates the conclusive nature of the positive test.

Likewise the chance of a negative test failing to identify a truly anaemic patient compared to correctly ruling out a healthy patient to not have anaemia is only 0.18. A higher LR+ and a lower LR– indicates better characteristic of a test. In this case study we have used the cut-off levels of serum ferritin as <60 mmol/l or ≥60 mmol/l to indicate positive or negative test results, respectively. What if we decide to change this cut-off level? Say if we increase the cut-off to 70 mmol/l, our test identifying true anaemic cases will increase (sensitivity will increase) but with a trade-off of decreased ability to rule out the true negatives (or specificity). This leads to one of the most asked questions: 'Which cut-off level is the best?' Receiver operator characteristic (ROC) curves will allow us to identify the ideal cut-off levels. Also, with different cut-off levels one could recompute LR+ and LR–, and evaluate what happens to the ability of the test to correctly rule in and rule out the patients and subjects.

Figure 7.2 Test results

		Iron deficiency anaemia (confirmed cases)	
		Present	*Absent*
Diagnostic test (serum ferritin)	Positive <60 mmol/l	250(*a*)	25(*b*)
	Negative ≥60 mmol/l	50(*c*)	425(*d*)

Sensitivity = $a/(a + c)$ = 250/(250 + 50) = 83%
Specificity = $d/(b + d)$ = 425/(25 + 425) = 94%
PV+ = $a/(a + b)$ = 250/(250 + 25) = 91%
PV– = $d/(c + d)$ = 425/(50 + 425) = 89%
LR+ = Sensitivity/(1 – Specificity) = 0.83/(1 – 0.94) = 13.8
LR– = (1 – Sensitivity)/Specificity = (1 – 0.83)/0.94 = 0.18

7.6.3 Receiver operator characteristics curves

When test results are continuous, several values of sensitivity and specificity are possible, depending on where the cut-off point is drawn. A receiver operator characteristic (ROC) curve is a graphical representation of the relationship between sensitivity and specificity at various cut-offs for any given test (Crichton 2002, Swets 1988, Fischer et al 2003), and is graphically represented in Figure 7.3.

The ROC curve can be used to determine the optimal cut-off point for the test. This curve is generated by first determining several different cut-offs and then calculating the sensitivity and specificity for each cut-off. The x-axis of the ROC curve is 1 minus the specificity (the false positives) and the y-axis is the sensitivity (the true positives). A diagonal line from the coordinates (0,0) to (1,1) on this graph represents a test that has no ability to discriminate those with or without the problem or condition (not sensitive nor specific). The closer a ROC curve gets to the left-hand corner (0,1), the better the test. The area under the curve is used to assess the ability of the test to discriminate. The perfect test has an area of 1.0 and a non-discriminating test has an area of 0.5.

Swets (1988) provides a 'rule of thumb' for interpreting ROC curves. He suggests that when the area under the curve is greater than 0.9 then the test has high accuracy and when it spans from 0.7 to 0.9, it has moderate accuracy. Areas of 0.5 to 0.7 have low accuracy and those of less than 0.5 are no more accurate than chance alone. Hanley and McNeil (1982) provide more in-depth discussion of ROC curves. O'Connell and Myers (2002) wrote a short article detailing their results of testing the Morse Fall scale. They describe its sensitivity and specificity in their population of patients in an Australian acute care setting. They also provide their ROC curve, demonstrating that the scale did not discriminate very well in their population. Directly following this article, Crichton (2002) provides a one-page 'information point' on ROC curves.

Figure 7.3 The receiver operator characteristic (ROC) curve

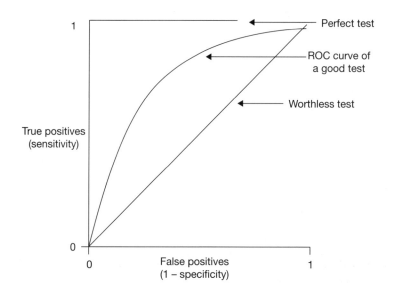

111

7.7 Is it possible to use this test with patients?

Clinicians want to know if a particular screening or diagnostic test should be used for a particular patient. Two things must be considered:
1. Is the test accurate?
2. Is it feasible to use?

Test accuracy is assessed by considering its sensitivity, specificity and likelihood ratio, and thus is quantitative in nature. Feasibility relates to whether the test is acceptable to people and whether it is cost-effective. Research to examine feasibility may be either quantitative or qualitative. Components of critical appraisal of quantitative evidence are provided below, followed by a discussion of qualitative evidence.

7.7.1 Critically appraising quantitative evidence

Just like any other kind of research, it is important to critically appraise studies that report on screening and diagnostic test accuracy (Jaeschke et al 1994a, Jaeschke et al 1994b). When reading journal articles about diagnostic tests, clinicians should consider several questions. These questions and their rationale are displayed in Table 7.1, and have been adapted from a variety of sources (Jaeschke et al 1994a, Jaeschke et al 1994b, Muir Gray 1997, Irwig et al 1994, Fischer et al 2003, Begg 1987).

Table 7.1 Criteria for appraising articles about screening and diagnostic tests

Question	Rationale
Were the setting and sample described in enough detail to understand their characteristics?	The reader has to consider how similar or different the sample is to their own population to make a decision on whether the test is applicable to their situation
Did the sample include a wide spectrum of subjects?	If only individuals at the severe end of the spectrum are included, then it is unclear if the test will distinguish those who are less severe but who could also benefit from treatment
If a diagnostic test, what reference standard was used?	If the standard itself is not accurate or appropriate for use with the test, then the study findings are questionable
If a diagnostic test, was the person who was responsible for administration of the test blinded to the reference standard results?	Knowledge of the reference standard results can influence diagnostic test interpretation; therefore bias can be introduced if the assessor was not blinded
Was the research protocol adhered to?	If some participants do not receive both the diagnostic test and the reference standard, then verification bias may be an issue
Was the sensitivity and specificity of the test identified?	These tests are used as a beginning step to assess the accuracy of the test itself
Was a likelihood ratio or receiver operator characteristic (ROC) curve provided?	These tests provide a more rigorous way of assessing the accuracy of the test itself and thus its utility
Were patients better off as a result of having the test?	There must be some benefits for spending the time and energy on testing

7.7.2 Critically appraising qualitative evidence

Studies that report on the accuracy of screening and diagnostic tests are quantitative in nature; however, qualitative research has the potential to play an important role in the use of these tests. In discussing the use of qualitative research to inform the evidence-based practitioner, Evans and Pearson (2001) suggest that qualitative evidence can be used to identify the appropriateness and feasibility of interventions. This perspective can be readily applied to the use of screening and diagnostic tests. Tests that are quick and easy to perform with minimal discomfort are likely to be more acceptable to individuals. Cost-effectiveness relates to the ability of the test to impact on the course of the problem or condition, when lead-time bias is taken into consideration. Treatments at this 'preclinical' phase must be more effective than treatments after the problem has emerged. Earlier in the chapter several principles for the use of tests were presented. These included the need for the problem or condition to be serious, to have beneficial treatment available, to have the resources for follow-up and for treatment to be acceptable. Qualitative research can provide valuable information in this area.

7.8 Conclusion

Screening and diagnostic tests are increasingly being used in nursing. Screening tests are designed to identify those at risk of developing some problem or condition, whereas diagnostic tests are designed to identify those with some problem or condition, before it is clinically evident. For these tests to be beneficial, first they need to be accurate, as demonstrated by their sensitivity and specificity. ROC curves and likelihood ratios provide more evidence of their accuracy. For tests to be beneficial, they also must result in better outcomes for individuals. That is, the test needs to result in some form of intervention that improves outcomes beyond what would be expected if the intervention were applied later, when the problem became evident.

7.9 Discussion questions

1. Differentiate between screening and diagnostic tests.
2. Discuss the criteria that guide decisions for using a screening or diagnostic test.
3. Describe methods used to assess the accuracy of screening and diagnostic tests.
4. Identify factors that may influence the sensitivity and specificity of a test.
5. Explain the benefits of reporting likelihood ratios and ROC curves.
6. Identify and discuss two major sources of bias in evaluating a screening test.

7.10 References

Anthony D, Clark M, Dallender J 2000 An optimization of the Waterlow score using regression and artificial neural networks. *Clinical Rehabilitation* 14(1):102–9.

Begg C B 1987 Biases in the assessment of diagnostic tests. *Statistics in Medicine* 6:411–23.

Crichton N 2002 Information point: receiver operating characteristic (ROC) curves. *Journal of Clinical Nursing* 11:136.

Cutson T M 1994 Falls in the elderly. *American Family Physician* 49:149–56.

Dujardin B, Van den Ende J, Van Gompel A et al 1994 Likelihood ratios: a real improvement for clinical decision making? *European Journal of Epidemiology* 10:29–36.

Eagle D J, Salama S, Whitman D et al 1999 Comparison of three instruments in predicting accidental falls in selected inpatients in a general teaching hospital. *Journal of Gerontological Nursing* 25(7):40–5.

Evans D, Pearson A 2001 Systematic reviews of qualitative research. *Clinical Effectiveness in Nursing* 5:111–19.

Fischer J E, Bachmann L M, Jaeschke R 2003 A readers' guide to the interpretation of diagnostic test properties: clinical example of sepsis. *Intensive Care Medicine* 29:1043–51.

Hanley J A, McNeil B J 1982 The meaning and use of the area under a receiver operating characteristic (ROC) curve. *Radiology* 143:29–36.

Hennekens C H, Buring J E 1987 *Epidemiology in medicine.* Little, Brown and Company, Boston.

Irwig L, Tosteson A N A, Gatsonis C et al 1994 Guidelines for meta-analyses evaluating diagnostic tests. *Annals of Internal Medicine* 120(8):667–76.

Jaeschke R, Guyatt G, Sackett D L 1994a How to use an article about a diagnostic test: are the results of the study valid? *Journal of the American Medical Association* 271(5):389–91.

Jaeschke R, Guyatt G, Sackett D L 1994b How to use an article about a diagnostic test: what are the results and will they help me in caring for my patients? *Journal of the American Medical Association* 271(9):703–7.

Kerr C, Taylor R, Heard G 1998 *Handbook of public health methods.* McGraw-Hill, Sydney.

Marx C M, Smith P G, Lowrie L H et al 1994 Optimal sedation of mechanically ventilated pediatric critical care patients. *Critical Care Medicine* 22:163–70.

Mercer L 1997 Falling out of favour. *Australian Nursing Journal* 4:27–9.

Muir Gray J A 1997 *Evidence-based Healthcare.* Churchill Livingstone, New York.

Newman T B, Browner W S, Cummings S R 2001 Designing studies of medical tests, in S B Hulley, W S Browner, D Grady et al (eds) *Designing clinical research: an epidemiologic approach,* 2nd edn. Lippincott Williams & Wilkins, Philadelphia.

O'Connell B, Myers H 2002 Research in brief: the sensitivity and specificity of the Morse Fall Scale in an acute care setting. *Journal of Clinical Nursing* 11:134–5.

Perell K L, Nelson A, Goldman R L et al 2001 Fall risk assessment measures: an analytic review. *Journal of Gerontology* 56A(12):M761–M766.

Ramsey M, Savage T, Simpson B, Goodwin R 1974 Controlled sedation with alphaxolone-alphadolone. *British Medical Journal* 2:656–9.

Swets J A 1988 Measuring the accuracy of diagnostic systems. *Science* 240:1285–93.

Woodbury M G, Houghton P E, Campbell K E, Keast D H 1999 Pressure ulcer assessment instruments: a critical appraisal. *Ostomy Wound Management* 45(5):42–55.

Young-McCaughan S, Miaskowski C 2001 Definition of and mechanism for opioid-induced sedation. *Pain Management Nursing* 2:84–97.

chapter ⑧

Outcomes for evidence-based nursing practice

Anne Chang

8.1 Learning objectives

After reading this chapter, you should be able to:

1. *explain the relationship between outcomes and evidence*
2. *distinguish between health and nursing outcomes in terms of sensitivity to nursing practice*
3. *identify the benefits of a system for classifying nursing outcomes*
4. *outline the purpose of including outcomes for feasibility, appropriateness and meaningfulness, as well as effectiveness, in planning to implement evidence*
5. *compare and contrast the validity of outcomes and the validity of tools for measuring outcomes, and*
6. *determine the main criteria to be considered in critically appraising outcomes for evidence of effectiveness.*

8.2 Introduction

Determining health-related outcomes that are sensitive to nursing interventions is crucial in providing evidence of the contribution nurses make in the healthcare system (Bond & Thomas 1991, Barriball & Mackenzie 1992, Pierce 1997, Maas 1996, Oermann & Floyd 2002). Both professional and managerial concerns underpin the focus on outcome measurement. In the former the emphasis is on demonstrating accountability through self and peer monitoring to ensure that patient outcomes are attained through high-quality care. While the initial focus in evidence-based systematic reviews was on outcomes demonstrating evidence of effectiveness, more comprehensive approaches to summarising research findings include health-related outcomes concerned with feasibility, appropriateness and meaningfulness, as well as effectiveness of nursing interventions (see www.joannabriggs.edu.au/related/sumari.php). The focus in the managerial perspective on outcomes is also on effectiveness, as well as on efficiency and reducing costs.

Lack of consistency in terms used to depict particular outcomes has led to confusion and discrepancy in measurement. Moorhead et al (2004) point to the many different outcomes developed for specific settings, which are unable to be used in other settings. Undertaking systematic reviews of research evidence is difficult with such diversity in depicting the results of nursing care and leads to fragmentation in the evidence base for nursing practice. The development of outcome classification systems is a step forward in clarifying the terminology used to depict outcomes, as in the work of the Nursing Outcomes Classification (NOC).

Highlighting those health-related outcomes that are sensitive to nursing interventions complements such classification systems and ultimately enables articulation of the nursing contribution to healthcare. The systematic review process requires rigorous appraisal of the quality and level of the evidence as depicted by the outcomes of each study included in the review.

8.3 What are outcomes?

This section provides a general definition of outcomes, and then defines 'health outcomes', followed by the more specific 'nursing or patient outcomes'. The link between outcomes and interventions is then briefly discussed.

8.3.1 General definition

While outcomes are defined as the consequences or end results, health outcomes refer to the consequences of an alteration in patients' health status or behaviour. The type of outcome generally identifies the nature of the process or action that led to the particular outcome. Accordingly, health and nursing outcomes refer to the result arising from preceding care and treatment (Bond & Thomas 1991), be it healthcare by a group of health professionals or care provided by nurses. Such care in the healthcare environment includes health promotion and preventative interventions.

A focus on outcomes and effectiveness in healthcare commenced in the early 1980s along with the orientation on determining the quality of care provided by healthcare services (Muir Gray 2001). However, over time limitations of an outcomes orientation have become evident. As well as treatment and/or care, additional factors such as individual differences, interrelationships, environment, illness severity and previous illnesses needed to be considered as influencing outcomes (Sidani & Braden 1998, Muir Gray 2001). Additionally the outcomes of an intervention can be both intended or planned for, as well as unintended, or unplanned and unexpected (Sidani & Braden 1998).

8.3.2 Health outcomes

Health outcomes are broader and more encompassing responses to interventions by any health professional. Thus nurses as well as other health professionals may contribute to the health status (Sidani & Braden 1998). The more traditional health outcomes of mortality, morbidity, adverse outcomes and length of stay have long been used to determine the effects of medical interventions. These outcomes are very broad and overarching indicators of the quality of care that focus on physical aspects and provide no real indication of the effects of the disease or treatment on individuals' lives (Oermann & Huber 1999). Such broad outcomes are unable to provide specific information on how the treatment affected the outcomes for individuals (Nolan & Mock 2000).

Hepworth (1997) points to the limitation of these traditional outcomes when used to determine the results of health promotion interventions and proposes three types of outcomes: health development outcomes; social health outcomes; and biomedical health outcomes. Such a typology assists in capturing the full range of outcomes provided within healthcare settings. However, for the purposes of determining evidence of effectiveness of nursing and midwifery interventions, the outcomes need to be sensitive and specific enough to detect whether a change has occurred or not.

8.3.3 Nursing or patient outcomes

Much of the research on nursing outcomes focuses on the results of nursing care on client/patient behaviour that is able to be observed (Spilsbury & Meyer 2001). Therefore the term 'nursing outcomes' can be seen as synonymous with patient/client outcomes. This is where potential for confusion arises, as the qualifier for the outcome (i.e. nurse or patient) would seem to indicate whose outcome is being referred to. Instead, Moorhead et al (2004) recommend that outcome labels should not be used to describe nurse behaviour. 'Outcomes of nursing' may be a preferred way of labelling these types of outcomes, as it would enable outcomes that refer to changes in nursing behaviour to be distinguished from changes brought about by nurses on patient outcomes (Griffiths 1995).

8.3.4 The link between outcomes and intervention

Determining the specific responses to particular interventions is the key to determining the evidence base for practice. More general outcomes provide a broad view of health status and overall quality of health, but are unlikely to indicate how a particular intervention 'worked'. In clinical practice and research it is important to consider how particular outcomes are related to the care or interventions provided. Research for developing clinically relevant knowledge needs to measure the outcome, the intervention and the influencing factors (Sidani & Braden 1998).

The link between the intervention and the outcomes needs to be clear to promote understanding of how the intervention produces change in the outcome. For example, a nursing intervention to promote self-esteem, which chooses functional ability as well as self-esteem as outcomes, may find no change in the first outcome but change in the second outcome that is more clearly related to the intervention (Chang 1999). The outcomes need to match the intervention (e.g. an educational intervention that uses information sessions, booklets and other media to provide patients and carers with requisite knowledge about diabetes does not necessarily lead to change in patient behaviour, but may well lead to improved levels of knowledge and understanding).

To change patient behaviour in regard to diabetes, other types of intervention are also needed in addition to education (e.g. interventions to promote self-management). Greater specificity in outcomes as in the preceding examples increases the likelihood of detecting a change that is due to the actual intervention and the resulting condition of the particular clients (Sidani & Braden 1998). See Table 8.1.

Table 8.1 Outcomes for self-esteem enhancement

Intervention	Outcome	Sensitive Yes/No
Self-esteem enhancement	Trait self-esteem	Depends if intervention is for long-term change in self-esteem
	State self-esteem	Yes, if for short-term
	Functional ability	No, although may be indirectly influenced by self-esteem level
Patient education	Adherence to medications	Unlikely unless skill component
	Knowledge of medications	Yes

Another example of the importance of being specific in matching the outcome to the intervention provided comes from the area of cardiac rehabilitation. Denollet (1993) identifies potential problems in assessing the psychological effect of cardiac rehabilitation. It is proposed that the outcome is not specific enough and thus unable to detect significant effects of the rehabilitation interventions. Furthermore, Denollet maintains that the outcome does not match the intervention, as many of the outcome measures reflect psychopathology and are inappropriate for most people with coronary heart disease. Rather the outcomes need to be related to the psychological effects of having this disease, such as reduced feelings of wellbeing and concerns about associated disabilities. Accordingly cardiac rehabilitation does not aim to change a person's psychopathology; it aims to assist individuals to adapt to their condition and adopt feelings and lifestyles that will promote wellbeing.

8.4 Classification of outcomes

The development of outcomes and systems for classifying them stems from early work on the evaluation of healthcare by such people as Florence Nightingale, Codman and Donabedian (Moorhead et al 2004). These developments gained momentum in the 1990s with greater emphasis being placed on healthcare effectiveness. Further refinement and development followed the recognition that nursing needed outcomes that would reflect the result of nursing care to demonstrate its contribution to healthcare.

8.4.1 Core outcomes

The core outcomes indicators for nursing identified by the American Nurses Association (ANA) (1995) for acute care include: mortality rate; length of stay; adverse incidents; complications; and patient satisfaction with nursing care. However, Moorhead et al (2004) point out that the breadth of these outcomes is more indicative of hospital or unit performance than of nursing care to individual patients.

Outcomes that are more specific for determining the effect of nursing have been developed by a number of different researchers since the 1970s. One example, by Marek (1990), demonstrates the main categories of outcome identified from a review of outcomes used in nursing research: physiologic; psychosocial; functional; behavioural; knowledge; home functioning; family strain; safety; symptom control; quality of life; goal attainment; patient satisfaction; utilisation of service; and nursing diagnosis resolution. Some of these categories remain quite broad and encompass many more specific outcomes (e.g. physiologic would comprise outcomes related to the main functions of the body).

Core outcomes with greater specificity for evaluating nurses' contribution to healthcare are those from the study by Moorhead et al (2004). They report on the evaluation of 174 outcome measures, after 16 pertaining to children were excluded, in 10 different healthcare settings, including hospital and community agencies. The 24 core outcomes found across settings were:

- *ambulation*—walking (1); comfort (2); communication ability (3); endurance (4); energy conservation (5); health-promoting behaviour (6); infection status (7); and information processing (8)
- *knowledge*—disease process (9)
- *knowledge*—medication (10); and mobility level (11)
- *nutritional status*—nutrient intake (12)
- *pain*—disruptive effects (13); and pain level (14)
- *participation*—healthcare decisions (15); quality of life (16); and rest (17)
- *safety behaviour*—fall prevention (18)
- *self-care*—activities of daily living (19)
- *self-care*—hygiene (20); sleep (21); and social support (22)
- *tissue integrity*—skin and mucous membranes (23); and vital signs status (24).

8.4.2 The Nursing Outcomes Classification (NOC)

The Nursing Outcomes Classification (NOC) has been developed as a comprehensive and standardised classification of patient outcomes that are responsive to nursing interventions (Moorhead et al 2004). Patient outcomes refer to outcomes for individuals, families and communities. A standardised system for labelling outcomes is necessary to enable the electronic capture and storage of this type of clinical information, which will enhance evaluation of effectiveness (Maas et al 2002).

The development of NOC commenced in 1991 with the clarification of the underlying conceptual and methodological issues. Outcomes were defined as: 'variable patient states that are influenced by nursing interventions to facilitate measurement of change' (Daly et al 1997:s84). From an initial list of 4500 patient outcomes, 282 nursing-sensitive patient outcomes and indicators were identified (Daly et al 1997). In 1997 the next round of development had resulted in 178 outcomes. The third edition of NOC resulted in 330 outcomes, which were classified into the seven domains of functional health, physiological health, psychosocial health, health knowledge and behaviour, perceived health, family health and community health (Moorhead, Johnson & Maas 2004). Across these seven domains are 31 classes or categories of outcome. For example, the outcome 'participation in healthcare decisions' is in the domain of 'health knowledge and behaviour', and in the class or category of 'health behaviour' (Moorhead et al 2004).

8.4.3 International Classification for Nursing Practice (ICNP)

Another classification system that assists in understanding the types of outcomes related to nursing is the International Classification for Nursing Practice (ICNP). However, the ICNP classifies more than outcomes; it also provides a system for categorising phenomena and actions. The ICNP was developed to provide 'a common language for describing nursing practice in order to improve communication among nurses and between nurses and others' (see www.icn.ch/icnpupdate.htm#Intro, 2004). Nursing outcomes are referred to in the ICNP classification as the results that are measured over time following nursing interventions that relate to particular nursing problems or diagnoses.

8.4.4 Types of outcomes

Outcomes will vary according to the different level of role of the nurse in decision making and initiation of care (Irvine et al 1998). When independent decisions are made by nurses about care, the changes to be measured in patient outcomes would relate to nurse assessment, nurse-initiated interventions and evaluation of care. In the dependent role of following the instructions of other health professionals, nurses would examine outcomes relating to side effects and other responses to treatment. In the interdependent role depicting the nurse as a team member the outcomes of relevance would be those concerned with the overall management and continuity of patient care (Irvine et al 1998). The interdependent role of the nurse is also referred to as the interdisciplinary role. Maas (1998), while recognising the willingness of nurses to be part of the team in patient care, also cautions nurses to be mindful of not losing sight of the contribution of the discipline of nursing to the work of the team.

8.4.4.1 Outcomes for feasibility, appropriateness, meaningfulness and effectiveness

Community and government demands for quality, legal and economic considerations have influenced the focus in the evidence-based literature on outcomes of effectiveness. However, an intervention may be found effective but considered to be impractical, inappropriate or meaningless to the patient, carer and/or health professional. Accordingly there is current recognition of the need to summarise evidence from other types of research that provide information on outcomes relating to the feasibility, appropriateness and meaningfulness of nursing interventions. A more encompassing approach to considering outcomes of nursing care is demonstrated by the Joanna Briggs Institute (JBI) FAME framework, which represents Feasibility, Appropriateness, Meaningfulness and Effectiveness (see www.joannabriggs.edu.au/related/sumari.php). Muir Gray (2001) identifies six outcomes, which are additional to those of effectiveness that can assist practitioners to decide on the intervention: equity; safety; patient satisfaction; cost-effectiveness; quality; and appropriateness.

8.5 Measuring outcomes

Measurement of the outcomes that result from interventions is essential in providing evidence of effectiveness. Measurement enables determining the extent to which the intervention resulted in both intended and unintended outcomes.

This section examines outcomes when planning intervention studies, focusing on the validity and reliability of those outcomes, and then aspects related to outcomes within a critical appraisal of studies of effectiveness.

In considering the validity in a study of effectiveness account needs to be taken of the *validity of the outcome* in determining whether an intervention was effective or not, as well as examining *the validity of a particular tool* to measure that outcome. Within the process of a systematic review any bias that may have occurred in the measurement of outcomes and the tools for measuring them has to be identified (JBIEBNM 2000). Issues that arise in the measurement of outcomes include distinguishing the nursing effect from other health professionals and the timing of the measurement of outcomes.

8.5.1 Validity of outcomes and outcome measures

Ensuring validity of outcomes is the first critical step before measuring outcomes of effectiveness. While numerous factors are important in determining the quality of studies, such as the design and execution of a study, the particular focus here is on the validity of outcomes and the associated tools (Sidani 1996). Sidani and Braden (1998) advocate greater attention to the selection of the outcomes for nursing research that are clinically relevant to ensure detection of the actual effect of an intervention, while controlling for the influence of other factors in the research setting. Valid outcomes will allow for the measurement of the specific changes or consequences that should follow the intervention. That is, the outcomes should accurately represent the intended effects of the intervention and be maximally responsive to the particular features of the intervention, and not be influenced by other factors within the study context (Sidani 1996). If the outcomes are not clearly related to the intervention then it would be difficult to establish their validity.

An example of the link between outcomes and interventions is the six NOC outcomes from the community health nursing setting, which were found to have content validity in a study of community health nurses (Head et al 2003). The six outcomes deemed appropriate for determining the effectiveness of community health nursing intervention were:
- *self-care*—activities of daily living (1); and instrumental activities of daily living (2)
- *treatment behaviour*—illness or injury (3)
- *knowledge*—health promotion (4), and
- *caregiver performance*—direct care (5); and caregiver physical health (6).

The choice of appropriate outcomes should be based on the aim and theoretical underpinnings of the nursing intervention being tested. Once the validity of the outcomes has been established, then the tools for measuring these outcomes need to be identified. The quality and appropriateness of the measurement of those outcomes has a direct impact on the strength of the evidence for a particular intervention. An example of the theoretical connection between intervention and outcomes as well as tools can be seen in the field of promoting exercise in older adults. Theories about self-efficacy and behaviour and previous research found that expectations about exercise influenced older adults' participation in exercise programs. Based on this theory and research, Resnick et al (2001) developed the Outcome Expectation for Exercise (OEE) Scale for use with older adults.

If inappropriate outcomes are selected, the actual changes that occur will be undetected resulting in invalid conclusions (Sidani & Braden 1998). A very effective intervention may have been carried out but the effectiveness may not be recognised as effective due to the use of inappropriate outcomes. An example is when studies of interventions to enhance self-esteem are implemented to newly admitted stroke patients. The type of self-esteem experienced by such individuals is more situational and changeable (state self-esteem) compared to the long-term personality trait type of self-esteem. Accordingly, lack of preciseness in the definition of self-esteem in such a situation may result in choosing an outcome of trait self-esteem and using a trait self-esteem measure such as the Rosenberg Self-esteem Scale (RSES) (Rosenberg 1965). It would therefore not be surprising if the trait self-esteem tool failed to detect any change and the intervention was deemed ineffective. The intervention for state self-esteem would differ from the intervention needed to change trait self-esteem, which would have to be particularly strong and longer term to change a person's enduring way of perceiving self. Strickland (1997) recognises this problem in the related area of anxiety, indicating that trait measures should be seen as a person's characteristic and that state measures that can detect change over time should be used.

In another example the absence of significant improvement in self-esteem (RSES) following a four-week intervention of hope instillation may have been due to the use of an inappropriate outcome such as trait self-esteem (Tollett & Thomas 1995). It is unlikely that a four-week intervention would change a person's personality trait of self-esteem. In another study a possible mismatch between interventions and outcomes may be the reason why exercise did not lead to self-esteem (RSES) improvements in an experimental group of breast cancer survivors compared to the control group (Segar et al 1998). The theoretical link between exercise and trait self-esteem would need to have been established for trait self-esteem to be a valid outcome for an exercise intervention.

8.5.2 Issues in the measurement of outcomes

Issues arising in regard to the measurement of patient outcomes include *sensitivity of the outcome measures, distinguishing the nursing contribution* from others in the healthcare team and the most appropriate *timing* for the measurement to occur.

8.5.2.1 Sensitivity of outcomes measures

Sensitivity adds a further dimension to the issue of validity by addressing two aspects of sensitivity—the accuracy in detecting change in the outcome and the responsiveness of the outcome measure (Sidani & Braden 1998). Sensitivity and specificity in terms of screening programs or diagnostic tools will not be discussed here, but rather the focus will be on the sensitivity in selecting the most appropriate outcomes to be used to measure the effectiveness of an intervention.

Accuracy in regard to sensitivity refers to the ability of a tool to detect real changes in outcome measures that are due to the intervention. One example is the outcomes used to determine the effectiveness of smoking cessation interventions. Self-report of quitting is one outcome that will be subject to the usual biases and thus inaccuracies found in any self-report. Biochemical validation of such reports provides a more accurate outcome measure for determining the effectiveness of a smoking cessation intervention.

The responsiveness of an outcome measure means that it is able to detect the smallest amounts of change in an outcome (Nolan & Mock 2000, Strickland 1997). Sensitivity measures should be able to detect differences due to the intervention rather than the individual differences among subjects (Sidani & Braden 1998) in the outcome between experimental and control groups.

An example of the sensitivity of outcomes to detect treatment effects is demonstrated in the study by Denollet (1993). The findings from three outcome measures for psychological state in patients undergoing cardiac rehabilitation were compared. Two of the measures were standard measures for psychological wellbeing, the State Anxiety Inventory (STAI) and the Symptom Check List (SCL–90) (Derogatis et al 1973). The third measure of psychological state was the Heart Patients Psychological Questionnaire (HPPQ) (Erdman et al 1986). The HPPQ was found to be more sensitive than the other two tools in detecting changes from the cardiac rehabilitation program for patients with high and low baseline scores. The other two instruments indicated smaller amounts of change than the HPPQ for those with higher baseline scores and detected no changes for those with a low baseline HPPQ. The author points to the matching of the HPPQ with the intervention of cardiac rehabilitation in contrast to the STAI and SCL–90 and the tool's sensitivity to small changes in the outcome.

8.5.2.2 Distinguishing the nursing contribution

Given the current emphasis on the interdisciplinary nature of much of nursing care it is necessary to consider the ability of outcomes and tools to distinguish the effect of nursing interventions from the interventions of other health professionals (Strickland 1997). The more general the outcome the more likely it is that the intervention was provided by a group of health professionals (Maas et al 1996). This has yet to be achieved in the area of stroke rehabilitation. The systematic review by the Stroke Unit Trialists' Collaboration (2004) reports on the effectiveness of stroke units in the care of stroke patients with one-year outcomes demonstrating benefits to patients in terms of mortality, independence and home living. While it is of benefit to patients that it is known that dedicated stroke units produce better outcomes than general wards, this review provides no information about the particular intervention/s that contributed to these outcomes. Identification of the contribution of nurses to stroke patients' outcomes would need to focus on the particular activities of the nurse, which could include the promotion of independence in daily activities and the enhancement of self-esteem. Effectiveness of aspects of the medical management of stroke patients has been established—for example, in the benefit of antiplatelet therapy (Sandercock et al 2004).

More research in areas of nursing practice will help to provide evidence of the contribution of nurses. Strickland (1997) proposes that nurses should focus on more positive outcomes than on the disease-and-cure focus, which has a more negative orientation to outcomes. Identifying the contribution of nursing within team approaches can be achieved to some extent through the selection of appropriate outcomes. Thus the outcomes that nurses should emphasise are those related to health promotion, enhancing health status, and promoting self-care and knowledge.

8.5.2.3 Timing for measuring the outcome

There are no hard and fast rules about the timing for measuring outcomes in effectiveness research; it is the nature of the intervention, outcome and disease that informs the researcher on the most suitable times. The timing and number of occasions for measurement will vary according to the selected outcomes and interventions being tested, as well as on the healthcare condition (Strickland 1997). The outcome may be measured immediately following an intervention, or hours, days or weeks after the intervention (Nolan & Mock 2000).

The precise timing of the measurement of outcomes will be dependent on when the intervention should achieve the aimed effects (Strickland 1997). The time taken for the outcome to come to fruition can vary with some effects being evident in a few days and others taking weeks or months. Sustainability of the effect of an intervention may also be important and thus require repeated measurement (Sidani & Braden 1998). Reviews of effectiveness of interventions take account of the timing of the outcomes in determining the validity of the conclusions of the study (Sidani & Braden 1998). Failure to detect changes in outcomes following interventions may be due to incorrect timing of the measurement of outcomes (Kirchhoff & Dille 1994).

8.5.3 Baseline measurement of outcomes

Effectiveness research would normally include measurement of outcomes prior to the implementation of the intervention being tested as well as following the intervention. A typical example is the measurement of knowledge and understanding prior to the commencement of a program of patient teaching. The initial measurement provides information on the level of the outcome of interest (e.g. knowledge and understanding) and enables examination of the equivalence of the study groups (e.g. comparing the baseline knowledge of the intervention group with the knowledge of a control group). Non-equivalence of groups at baseline on the effectiveness outcomes will need to be accounted for in data analysis for determining the effectiveness of the intervention.

8.5.4 Postintervention measurement of outcomes

The timing for the postintervention measurement is important and should be guided by the underlying theory of the intervention and health condition, as well as by the time taken to carry out the intervention. The intervention may take hours, days or weeks to take effect and thus the measurement needs to match the timing of effectiveness. Additionally the effectiveness of an intervention may be determined by its ability to sustain the outcome, so that repeated measurement may be needed.

In the case of patient teaching (e.g. on preoperative preparation one week before surgery), it is likely that the level of knowledge measured immediately following completion of a patient education program would be a significant outcome. However, it may also be important to see if the knowledge level can be maintained and thus a further episode of measurement might occur in one week upon admission.

However, when the intervention is conducted over a few weeks or months, measurement of the outcome during the intervention may also be undertaken. As there are likely to be different sections in long education programs, the outcomes may vary and measurement could occur at different times to match the focus of the intervention at that time. An example is the antenatal education provided to women throughout their pregnancy. The purposes of antenatal education can include learning about body changes throughout pregnancy, preparing for labour and parenting. The measurement of each of these sections will be determined by the timing of the section of the education program. Chronologically these three sections of an antenatal education program represent different time points throughout the pregnancy and childbirth, and thus identify the most appropriate time for determining the effectiveness of each part of the education program.

In a study examining the effects of a psychosocial intervention for stroke patients the postintervention outcomes were measured at two weeks and three months after patients' admission to a stroke rehabilitation hospital. The first postintervention episode of data collection occurred at two weeks following admission to ensure that patients had had sufficient exposure to the new intervention (Chang 1999). The second postintervention data collection at three months was for determining the longer term effects of the intervention and was guided by past research indicating when improvements for stroke patients should have occurred (Chang 1999).

8.5.5 Reliability

Once the validity of an outcome measure has been established attention is then directed to the reliability or consistency of the findings from the use of the outcome tools. In choosing the most appropriate tools attention is needed on the internal consistency of a tool as measured by Cronbach's alpha coefficient. This coefficient indicates the extent to which the items comprising a tool measure the same construct (Sidani & Braden 1998). The level of alpha coefficient that is seen as acceptable is 0.80 or higher; however, 0.70 is acceptable particularly for a new instrument (Nolan & Mock 2000). If a tool on anxiety has items of anxiety and also items related to social support, then the internal consistency could be expected to be lower than if the tool contained only anxiety items. As well as informing the researcher when choosing a tool to measure the study outcomes, reliability of the tools used in the study also needs to be established. This will give information on the reliability within the current study subjects.

Reliability also provides information about the level of error or 'fluctuations in the measure scores that are unrelated to the characteristic being measured' (Sidani & Braden 1998:154). Such fluctuations can be due to many factors including chance, the method and consistency that the tool is administered to the study subjects, the clarity of the tool and its instructions for administration, fatigue of the study subjects and the time of day. Such error or inconsistency in a tool results in greater variability of the results of the tool, which makes it difficult to detect the effectiveness of the intervention.

If there are to be a number of data collectors then the interrater reliability of the outcome measure needs to be determined (Sidani & Braden 1998). Clarification of the processes used in data collection by each of the raters should occur if the interrater reliability is below the accepted level of 0.75 (Portney & Watkins 2000).

125

8.5.6 Critical appraisal of outcomes for evidence of effectiveness

Nurse clinicians are keen to find evidence of effectiveness for interventions to be applied within their practice. When a systematic review reports positive changes in the outcome in well-conducted studies, the clinician will have greater confidence in using the tested intervention. The level of evidence will be stronger if the majority of studies in the systematic review are of good quality research and have findings in support of the intervention. Variation in results with some outcomes indicating effectiveness and others that the intervention is ineffective or makes no difference will weaken the level of evidence and thus the confidence in applying the results in the care of patients.

Assessing the quality of individual studies included within a systematic review in terms of outcomes involves checking whether the outcomes have been included and described for each study (JBIEBNM 2000, Grimshaw et al 2003). In turn, critical appraisals of systematic reviews contain as part of the methodology (as in Ch 5) quality assessment of the methods used in the study. In terms of outcomes the criteria for quality appraisal include whether the method for assessing outcomes was clearly defined and described, and whether the person assessing the outcome was blinded to the allocation of subjects to the treatment or the control group (Oxman 1994).

Reviewing the quality of the evidence of effectiveness for an intervention also requires examination of the number of outcomes, the size of the effect of the intervention on the outcome and the level of confidence in generalising the findings (Muir Gray 2001).

8.5.7 Number of outcomes

Several outcomes may be used to determine the effectiveness of an intervention, which then requires that health professionals determine if they all are beneficial or if some have adverse outcomes. If there is a mixture of beneficial and harmful outcomes then a process of weighing up the benefits while bearing in mind the harmful effects is needed (Muir Gray 2001). Consider the example of providing patient education on impending surgery.

One outcome could be that there was an increase in the level of knowledge of the patients; however, there was also an increase in the anxiety level in the experimental group, no doubt due to having more to worry about. The possible adverse effect of anxiety for a patient undergoing surgery needs to be compared to the beneficial effect of increased knowledge. It may be that the patient education intervention could be used but adjusted in some way to reduce the anxiety.

8.5.8 Effect size and confidence intervals

The size of the effect of an intervention refers to the extent to which the outcomes demonstrate the occurrence of an event (Cohen 1992). Cohen has developed standardised effect sizes to represent small, medium and large effect sizes. Interventions with large effect sizes usually require only small samples to detect differences between the experimental and control groups. The converse is true for interventions with small effect sizes. Numerous systematic reviews and discursive papers have pointed to the inadequacy of many nursing intervention studies due to the inadequacy of the sample size to detect a difference between the treatment and control groups. However, a small effect size is not the only reason for the failure to find an effect of the treatment; there could be many explanations including that the intervention was not strong enough to produce changes in the outcome. Additionally the effect size does not necessarily indicate the clinical significance of study findings; this would need to be determined by clinicians (Burns 2000).

Many intervention studies in nursing have been designated as having a medium effect size, but where possible the effect size should be more precisely determined from previous studies and with consideration to an effect size that will be clinically meaningful. An example of determining the effect size for a study testing the effectiveness of a nursing intervention is the study by Cheung et al (2003). These researchers used the finding of a medium effect size from an earlier pilot study (Cheung et al 2001) to estimate the sample size required for their main study on the effectiveness of progressive muscle relaxation on the outcome of anxiety of patients undergoing stoma surgery. The main study found a significantly lower level of anxiety for the experimental group.

Typically in meta-analyses of pooled individual studies, effect size is represented by the odds ratio. This is the ratio of the odds of the two groups. The odds are calculated for each group and refer to the number with a positive outcome divided by the number with a negative outcome (Altman 2000). Conventionally the ratio refers to the treatment group divided by the control group. For example, the odds of the experimental group having an improvement in knowledge following education are 70/30 (70 had increased knowledge and 30 did not) = 2.33. The odds of the control group having an improvement in knowledge following education are 32/40 (32 had increased knowledge and 40 did not) = 0.8. Therefore, the odds ratio is 2.33/0.8 = 2.92.

Confidence intervals for research results refer to the probability that the findings from a sample can be generalised to the population. The use of confidence levels is recommended for sample findings instead of levels of significance (p) to provide a range within which an intervention may be found effective for a population (Gardner & Altman 2000).

A forest plot is used to graphically present the odds ratio and confidence intervals for findings from different studies included in a systematic review or meta-analysis (Altman 2000). See the example of fictitious data in Figure 8.1.

8.5.9 Benefit and relevance

Additional factors to be considered in assessing the outcomes for evidence-based healthcare are the balance between benefit and harm, as well as the relevance of the findings for local populations and for individual patients. Outcomes may reveal that an intervention did more harm than good, or alternatively was of greater benefit than harm to the subjects. A third position regarding benefit is that the outcomes had no effect—that is, they were neither harmful nor beneficial (Muir Gray 2001).

Such considerations help the clinician in deciding whether to use the intervention. In the case of patient preoperative education, it may be that the education was deemed to be of greater benefit than the minimal increase in anxiety, and so the education program would be adopted by the clinical nurse. However, if the outcomes revealed a high level of anxiety with moderate to low knowledge gains for a specific patient group, then the education program would be judged as unsuitable.

Figure 8.1 Odds ratio and confidence intervals

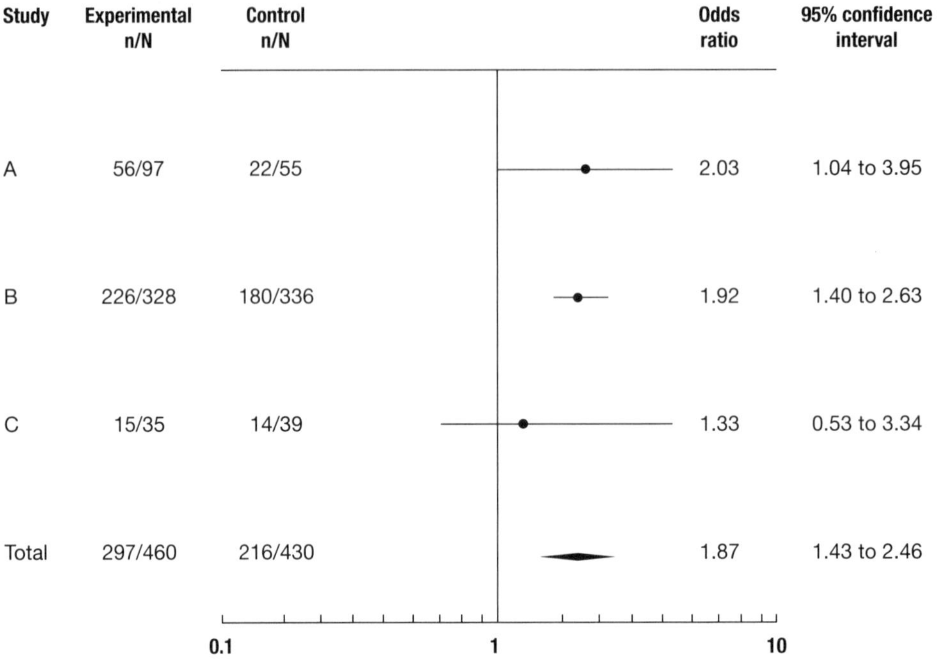

Study	Experimental n/N	Control n/N		Odds ratio	95% confidence interval
A	56/97	22/55		2.03	1.04 to 3.95
B	226/328	180/336		1.92	1.40 to 2.63
C	15/35	14/39		1.33	0.53 to 3.34
Total	297/460	216/430		1.87	1.43 to 2.46

0.1   1   10

The relevance of the intervention for adoption into particular clinical settings requires comparisons between the study population and the population where the intervention is being considered. Differences in the resources, demographics, values and beliefs may render the intervention unsuitable in the new setting. Furthermore at the level of the individual for whom the intervention is being considered the same type of comparisons would be needed in considering adoption of an intervention. These qualitative elements in assessing the applicability of an intervention in terms of the effectiveness outcomes are also addressed in Chapter 6, which discusses the evidence for the feasibility, appropriateness and meaningfulness of an intervention.

8.6 Conclusion

Evidence for nursing practice is based on the evaluation of outcomes that are sensitive to the care provided by nurses. A recognised system for labelling and classifying the outcomes resulting from nursing care is essential for improving consistency in the language that identifies nurses' contribution to healthcare. Such consistency is also necessary for building the body of evidence and knowledge underpinning nursing practice. This chapter has focused on outcomes of effectiveness, as evidence of this type provides direction for nurses and policy makers. However, outcomes related to the feasibility, appropriateness and meaningfulness also need to be considered in adopting a particular nursing intervention.

8.7 Discussion questions

1. Rate the extent to which the outcomes in Table 8.2 would be sensitive enough to detect changes in nursing care provided.

Table 8.2 Outcomes

Nursing care	Outcome	Very	Moderately	Somewhat	Not at all
Patient education on diabetes (newly diagnosed)	Coping with changes in life due to newly diagnosed disease				
Progressive muscle relaxation	Reduced anxiety				
Promoting self-esteem	Improved functional ability				
Health promotion on benefits of abstinence from smoking	Reduction in lung cancer rates				

2. For a systematic review, read S L Norris 2001 Effectiveness of self-management training in type 2 diabetes: a systematic review of randomized controlled trials. *Diabetes Care* 24(3):561–87. (The full-text article is available through CINAHL.) Critically appraise the outcomes from the review. Critical appraisal criteria for outcomes in the review include:
   —Were the methods for assessing outcomes clearly defined and described?
   —Was the assessor of the outcomes blinded to the allocation of subjects to the treatment or control group?
   Outcomes include:
   —knowledge
   —frequency and accuracy of self-monitoring of blood glucose
   —self-reported dietary habits, and
   —glycaemic control.
3. Consider how other types of evidence—feasibility, appropriateness and meaningfulness—might impact on the decision to change the type of mattresses used in a healthcare facility following the evidence of effectiveness below:

   Evidence of effectiveness shows that ordinary foam mattresses should not be used for patients at high risk of pressure sore development. Additionally evidence of effectiveness indicates that in order to reduce the incidence of pressure sores in such patients, mattresses with higher specification should be used (Cullum et al 2004).

8.8 References

Altman D G Clinical trials and meta-analyses, in D G Altman, D Machin, T N Bryant & M J Gardner 2000 *Statistics with confidence*, 2nd edn. British Medical Journal, Bristol.
Altman D G, Machin D, Bryant T N, Gardner M J 2000 *Statistics with confidence*, 2nd edn. British Medical Journal, Bristol.

American Nurses Association (ANA) 1995 *Nursing care report card for acute care.* American Nurses Publishing, Washington DC.

Barriball K L, Mackenzie A 1992 The demand for measuring the impact of nursing interventions: a community perspective. *Journal of Clinical Nursing* 1(4):207–12.

Bond S, Thomas L H 1991 Issues in measuring outcomes of nursing. *Journal of Advanced Nursing* 16:1492–502.

Burns K J 2000 Power and effect size: research considerations for the clinical nurse specialist. *Clinical Nurse Specialist* 14(2):61–8.

Chang A M 1999 Psychosocial nursing intervention to promote self-esteem and functional independence following stroke. Unpublished PhD dissertation, the Chinese University of Hong Kong.

Cheung Y L C, Molassiotis A, Chang A M 2001 A pilot study on the effect of progressive muscle relaxation training of patients after stoma surgery. *European Journal of Cancer Care* 10(2):107–14.

Cheung Y L, Molassiotis A, Chang A M 2003 The effect of progressive muscle relaxation training on anxiety and quality of life after stoma surgery in colorectal cancer patients. *Psycho-Oncology* 12(3):254–66.

Cohen J 1992 A power primer. *Psychological Bulletin* 112(1):155–9.

Conn V S 2001 Designing effective nursing interventions. *Research in Nursing & Health* 24(5):433–42.

Cullum N, Deeks J, Sheldon T A et al 2004 Beds, mattresses and cushions for pressure sore prevention and treatment (Cochrane Review), in *The Cochrane Library*, Issue 2, John Wiley & Sons, Chichester.

Daly J M, Maas M L, Johnson M 1997 Nursing outcomes classification: an essential element in data sets for nursing and health care effectiveness. *Computers in Nursing* 15(2 Suppl):s82–6.

Denollet J 1993 Sensitivity of outcome assessment in cardiac rehabilitation. *Journal of Consulting and Clinical Psychology* 61(4):686–95.

Derogatis L R, Lipman R S, Covi L 1973 SCL–90: an outpatient psychiatric rating scale—preliminary report. *Psychopharmacology Bulletin* 9:13–27.

Erdman R A, Duivenvoorden H J, Verhage F et al 1986 Predictability of beneficial effects in cardiac rehabilitation: a randomized clinical trial of psychosocial variables. *Journal of Cardiopulmonary Rehabilitation* 6:206–13.

Gamel C J 2001 A method to develop a nursing intervention: the contribution of qualitative studies to the process. *Journal of Advanced Nursing* 33(6):806–19.

Gardner M J, Altman D G Estimating with confidence, in D G Altman, D Machin, T N Bryant & M J Gardner 2000 *Statistics with confidence*, 2nd edn. British Medical Journal, Bristol.

Gillis A 1995 Exploring nursing outcomes for health promotion. *Nursing Forum* 30(2):5–12.

Griffiths P 1995 Progress in measuring nursing outcomes. *Journal of Advanced Nursing* 21(6):1092–100.

Grimshaw J, McAuley L M, Bero L A et al 2003 Systematic reviews of the effectiveness of quality improvement strategies and programmes. *Quality and Safety in Health Care* August, 12(4):298–303.

Guyatt G H, Osoba D, Wu A W et al 2002 Methods to explain the clinical significance of health status measures. *Mayo Clinic Proceedings* 77(4):371–84.

Head B J, Maas M, Johnson M 2003 Validity and community-health-nursing sensitivity of six outcomes for community health nursing with older clients. *Public Health Nursing* 20(5):385–98.

Hepworth J 1997 Evaluation in health outcomes research: linking theories, methodologies and practice in health promotion. *Health Promotion International* 12(3):233–8.

International Classification of Nursing Practice (ICNP) International Council of Nurses (ICN). Available at http://www/icn.ch/icnpupdate.htm.

Irvine D, Sidani S, McGillis Hall L 1998 Linking outcomes to nurses' roles in health care. *Nursing Economic$* 16(2):58–64, 87.

Joanna Briggs Institute for Evidence Based Nursing and Midwifery (JBIEBNM) 2000 *Appraising systematic reviews, changing practice* 1(1). Available at www.joannabriggs.edu.au/CP1.pdf, and viewed 20 April 2004.

Kirchhoff K T, Dille C A 1994 Issues in intervention research: maintaining integrity. *Applied Nursing Research* 7(1):32–46.

Maas M L 1998 Nursing's role in interdisciplinary accountability for patient outcomes. *Outcomes Management for Nursing Practice* 2(3):92–4.

Maas M, Johnson M, Moorhead S 1996 Classifying nursing-sensitive patient outcomes. *Image: The Journal of Nursing Scholarship* 28(4):295–301.

Maas M L, Reed D, Reeder K M et al 2002 Nursing outcomes classification: a preliminary report of field testing. *Outcomes Management* 6(3):112–19.

Marek K D 1990 Outcomes measurement in nursing. *Journal of Nursing Quality Assurance* 4:1–9.

Moorhead S, Johnson M, Maas M (eds) 2004 *Nursing Outcomes Classification (NOC)*, 3rd edn. Mosby, St Louis.

Muir Gray J A 2001 *Evidence-based healthcare: how to make health policy and management decisions*, 2nd edn. Churchill Livingstone, New York.

Nolan M T, Mock V 2000 *Measuring patient outcomes*. Sage Publications, Thousand Oaks.

Oermann M H, Floyd J A 2002 Outcomes research: an essential component of the advanced practice nurse role. *Clinical Nurse Specialist* 16(3):140–6.

Oermann M H, Huber D 1999 Patient outcomes: a measure of nursing's value. *American Journal of Nursing* 99(9):40–8.

Oxman A D 1994 Checklists for review articles. *British Medical Journal* 309(6955):648–51.

Pierce S F 1997 Nurse-sensitive health care outcomes in acute care settings: an integrative analysis of the literature ... reprinted from *Journal of Nursing Care Quarterly* 11(4):60–72. *Journal of Rehabilitation Outcomes Measurement* 1(6):39–47.

Portney L G, Watkins M P 2000 *Foundations of clinical research: applications to practice*, 2nd edn. Prentice Hall Health, Upper Saddle River.

Resnick B, Zimmerman S, Orwig D et al 2001 Model testing for reliability and validity of the Outcome Expectations for Exercise Scale. *Nursing Research* 50(5):293–9.

Rosenberg M 1965 *Society and the adolescent self-image*. Princeton University Press, Princeton.

Sandercock P, Gubitz G, Foley P, Counsell C 2004 Antiplatelet therapy for acute ischaemic stroke (Cochrane Review), in *The Cochrane Library*, Issue 1, John Wiley & Sons, Chichester.

Segar M L, Katch V L, Roth R S et al 1998 The effect of aerobic exercise on self-esteem and depressive and anxiety symptoms among breast cancer survivors. *Oncology Nursing Forum* 25(1):107–13.

Sidani S 1996 Methodological issues in outcomes research. *Canadian Journal of Nursing Research* 28(3):87–94.

Sidani S, Braden C J 1998 *Evaluating nursing interventions: a theory-driven approach*. Sage Publications, Thousand Oaks.

Spilsbury K, Meyer J 2001 Defining the nursing contribution to patient outcome: lessons from a review of the literature examining nursing outcomes, skill mix and changing roles. *Journal of Clinical Nursing* 10(1):3–14.

Strickland O L 1997 Challenges in measuring patient outcomes. *Nursing Clinics of North America* 32(3):495–512.

Stroke Unit Trialists' Collaboration 2004 Organised inpatient (stroke unit) care for stroke (Cochrane Review), in *The Cochrane Library*, Issue 1, John Wiley & Sons, Chichester.

Tollett J H, Thomas S P 1995 A theory-based nursing intervention to instill hope in homeless veterans. *Advances in Nursing Science* 18(2):76–90.

part four ◎——•

Implementing evidence in practice

chapter ⑨

Developing a culture of inquiry to sustain evidence-based practice

Sonya Osborne and Glenn Gardner

9.1 Learning objectives

After reading this chapter, you should be able to:

1. *describe important features of an evidence-based culture and assess your own organisation in relation to these features*
2. *discuss barriers that impede development of an evidence-based culture of inquiry and identify the presence of any of these barriers in your own organisation, and*
3. *identify a range of strategies for developing and sustaining an evidence-based culture of inquiry, particularly those that may work in your organisation.*

9.2 Introduction

> *Culture does not change because we desire to change it. Culture changes when the organization is transformed; the culture reflects the realities of people working together every day*
> *(Hesselbein 2002:2).*

Evidence-based practice (EBP) is having a significant effect on the health service environment. It constructs a language that bridges the healthcare disciplines and the clinical and managerial components of health services. Most experienced clinicians in nursing, medicine and allied health now recognise that the contemporary healthcare environment calls for our practice to be justified by sound, credible evidence. There is pressure on all clinicians to accommodate innovation, while at the same time ensuring their practice is effective, safe and efficient (Forbes & Griffiths 2002). Consequently, EBP in healthcare is having a profound effect on nursing and the way we think about nursing.

There are many available models for research utilisation that are dependent on organisational strategies for change. This chapter describes the relationship between organisation and culture and explores the notion of evidence-based cultural change that requires change at both macro and micro levels (i.e. change at the systems level and change at the level of the individual clinician). We begin this chapter with a clear conception of what we mean by EBP and what we mean by 'culture'.

9.3 Evidence-based practice in healthcare

EBP has been thoroughly defined in Chapter 1. In summary, EBP is making clinical decisions using the best available evidence, in conjunction with clinical expertise, and judgment and knowledge of the patient. Essentially, EBP is about reducing uncertainty in clinical care leading to efficient and effective service delivery. It is about asking questions of our practice, systematically searching for answers to these questions, applying the best possible evidence from this search at the clinical interface and then evaluating the effect of this evidence-informed care.

However, evidence-based decision making is not as easy as following a five- or six-step recipe. Firstly, clinicians are not born with the skills to be evidence-based practitioners. Secondly, the 'evidence' is, quite often, inaccessible, unreadable, invalid, not available, not applicable or lacking in quality (Bryar et al 2003, Funk et al 1991, Kajermo et al 1998, Miller & Messenger 1978, Parahoo 2001, Retsas 2000). Although healthcare organisations pay lip-service to promoting and supporting the idea of EBP, few provide the infrastructure, resources, support and incentives necessary to develop and sustain a culture of inquiry.

First, there is lack of organisational support to develop EBP and research utilisation knowledge and skills of nurse clinicians, and, secondly (in the absence of evidence), there is lack of organisational support to generate nurse-initiated evidence for practice through the conduct of research (Tranmer et al 1998). Supporting an organisational culture of inquiry happens in a cultural environment made up of individual clinicians and subgroups of individual clinicians, each with their own values, beliefs, assumptions and behaviours. Therefore, before we can expect an organisational cultural change we must first effect an attitudinal change in the individual clinician.

9.4 Culture and organisation in healthcare

In this chapter, we will take the anthropological view instead of the positivist view in defining what we mean by culture—that is, a discussion based on the premise that an organisation does not *have* a culture, it *is* a culture. A common expression defining culture in the healthcare environment is 'culture is the way we do things around here'. Others have defined culture more formally as:

> ... a pattern of shared basic assumptions that the group learned
> as it solved its problems of external adaptation and internal
> investigation, that has worked well enough to be considered valid
> and, therefore, to be taught to new members as the correct way to
> perceive, think, and feel in relation to those problems
> (Schein 1992:12).

However, in any organisation, the organisational culture also contains a number of subcultures that ascribe to a pattern of basic assumptions based on a shared perspective. In healthcare those shared perspectives can be based on discipline (e.g. nurses or medical doctors), gender, age, geographical location (e.g. ward or unit, acute facility or community outreach clinic), experience (e.g. novice nurses or expert nurses) or specialty field (e.g. acute care or critical care; orthopaedics or oncology). By making organisation synonymous with culture, cultural change involves altering or transforming the basic assumptions of the organisation. If the basic assumptions of the subcultures make up the organisational culture, then cultural change will have to begin with the subcultures and, more basically, with the individuals that make up the subcultures. Given that definitions determine actions, thoughts and perceptions (Bate 1994:9), we must conceptualise an evidence-based culture, or more aptly, *a culture of inquiry*, before we can discuss and recognise a 'cultural change'.

9.5 What is a culture of inquiry?

In order to transform organisational culture to one that values EBP, it is necessary to have a clear idea of what a culture of inquiry looks like. A culture of inquiry is a culture that supports clinicians to make healthcare decisions that are based upon finding and using the best available evidence and combining that with their clinical expertise and their knowledge of the patient to guide decision making in healthcare. An organisation that promotes a culture of inquiry must:
* develop clinicians who are capable of using the evidence-based process in their clinical practice
* provide resources for clinicians to be evidence-based practitioners, and
* give clinicians the authority to participate collaboratively in healthcare decisions and effect change in their clinical practice based on best available evidence.

Learning has been described as being on a continuum, which, if reinforced over time, will lead to permanent changes in behaviour (Webb et al 1996). Thus, a culture of inquiry is a learning culture that encourages interrogation of practice by providing the necessary resources to formulate questions, search for answers and evaluate the answer in practice. Such a culture recognises the value of research and the integration of research findings into practice by providing the necessary infrastructure, resources, support and incentives to enable nurse clinicians to fully engage in the EBP agenda.

Healthcare occurs in a multidisciplinary and multidimensional environment. Therefore, a culture of inquiry tolerates diversity and promotes true collaboration in the decision-making process on issues regarding patient care. Such a culture also has particular attributes associated with a participative management, such as a flat versus hierarchical management framework and decentralised administration (Havens & Vasey 2003). Organisational strategies that enhance nurse involvement in decision making provide nurses with a voice in both patient care decisions and in nursing work decisions. Such involvement in decision making has implications for positive patient outcomes (Havens & Vasey 2003), such as lower patient morbidity and mortality (Aiken et al 1994, Baggs et al 1999), shorter mean length of stay (Aiken et al 1999), and fewer patient complaints (Havens 2001).

In addition to valuing collaboration and involvement in decision making, a culture of inquiry values and supports autonomy and authority in decision making in areas of expertise. Autonomy has been defined as 'an individual's ability to independently carry out the responsibilities of the position without close supervision' (Blanchfield & Biordi 1996:43). Authority has been defined as 'sanctioned or legitimate power to make decisions' (Blanchfield & Biordi 1996:43). Thus, a culture of inquiry recognises the legitimate authority of nurse clinicians, values professional nurse autonomy and encourages nurse involvement in healthcare decision making, thus providing support for change and innovation in practice.

There are benefits to having a culture of inquiry for both patients and nurses. It was demonstrated nearly two decades ago that patients who are the recipients of nursing care that is based on research have better outcomes. Heater et al (1988) conducted a meta-analysis of nurse-conducted experimental research and found that patients who are the recipients of research-based nursing interventions can expect 28% better outcomes than patients who receive standard nursing care. This early study supports the assumption that engagement in the EBP and research agenda improves patient outcomes.

Benefits to nurses working in an organisation that values EBP and nurses' contribution to healthcare has also been demonstrated in the literature. Several authors reported strong associations between autonomous decision making in clinical practice, job satisfaction and perceived productivity in organisations where the nurse leader values education and professional development of all nurses (Kramer & Schmalenberg 2003a, 2003b, Scott et al 1999). EBP is a great equaliser because the role of authority and opinion is no longer a sufficient basis for decisions about healthcare (Osborne & Gardner 2004). Rather, rules of evidence take precedence in clinical decision making (Osborne & Gardner 2004).

Later in this chapter, we will describe two different systems designed to nurture a learning culture that values research and translation of research into practice, diversity and collaboration, and autonomous decision making in order to develop and sustain a culture of inquiry, namely Magnet Hospitals and Practice Development Units.

9.6 Development towards a culture of inquiry

Gaining and maintaining commitment to organisational change is critical to enhancing the chances of a successful change towards a culture of inquiry. Since culture has been defined as a pattern of basic assumptions and values that an organisation shares, transforming to a culture of inquiry requires a change in the pattern of these basic assumptions and values. As an organisation is transformed to a culture of inquiry, clinical practice once guided by 'that's the way we do it around here' or 'that's the way we were told to do it' is replaced with clinical practice guided by the more questioning imperative of 'what's the evidence for that?'.

However, changing to a culture of inquiry can be problematic. Without simultaneous change at both the macro (organisation) level and micro (nurse clinician) level, cultural change will not be sustainable. Change in the culture of an organisation requires commitment to change by the individual members of the organisation's subcultures. However, to gain and maintain this commitment to change, the organisation must fully support its individual members throughout the change. Organisational support for a culture of inquiry is required to remove identified barriers to research utilisation, to build capacity to engage in the EBP agenda, and to encourage and support innovation in practice by recognising and supporting authority and autonomy for clinicians to effect practice change.

9.6.1 Removal of well-identified barriers

Research is still perceived by most nurse clinicians as external to practice and implementing research findings into practice is often difficult. Barriers to research utilisation by nurses have been discussed in the international nursing literature for the past three decades and are well documented in the literature (Bryar et al 2003, Funk et al 1991, Kajermo et al 1998, Miller & Messenger 1978, Parahoo 2001, Retsas 2000). In 1978, the most frequent problems encountered when trying to put research findings in place included:
1. inability to obtain research findings in one's own area of interest
2. the time and costs involved in implementing research
3. resistance to change in the work setting
4. lack of relevance of the findings
5. lack of understanding or agreement with conclusions, and
6. lack of rewards for implementation (Miller & Messenger 1978).
Although the quantity and quality of nursing research has improved since then, the use of research findings in practice remains low. In 1991, Funk et al (1991) found the two greatest barriers reported by nurses were 'nurses not feeling they had enough authority to change patient care procedures' and 'insufficient time on the job to implement new ideas'. Both are barriers of the organisational setting (Funk et al 1991). Moreover, most of the other barriers in the 'top 10 list' were those related to the organisational setting, including lack of cooperation and support from physicians, other staff and administration, inadequate facilities for implementation, and insufficient time to read research (Funk et al 1991). Barriers reported in the past vary little from barriers reported today. In general, aspects of the organisational setting and aspects of the research itself continue to represent the greatest problem areas. Lack of time to read and apply findings, lack of organisational and peer support, and lack of authority to change practice continue to rank highest in the list (Bryar et al 2003, Kajermo et al 1998, Parahoo 2001, Retsas 2000). To achieve successful cultural change towards a culture of inquiry, organisations must recognise these barriers and put strategies in place to reduce or eliminate them.

9.6.2 Capacity building in evidence-based practice and research utilisation

Difficulty in not only understanding but also accepting research findings is widespread (Bryar et al 2003, Funk et al 1991, Kajermo et al 1998, Miller & Messenger 1978, Parahoo 2001, Retsas 2000), and presents a serious challenge for the promotion of EBP in nursing. This is an issue not easily solved and in part is related to the nursing culture. Nursing is an old profession. Our beginnings are steeped in rituals, traditions and folklore. Despite the fact that nursing has changed in recent years and the *context* of nursing practice has changed dramatically, for too many nurses these rituals, traditions and folklores persist

(Holland 1993, O'Callaghan 2001, Strange 2002, Winslow 1998). This creates an environment that resists change, does not question and does not look to science to inform practice. In this environment research skills will not be valued. In conjunction with this historical cultural background is the varying quality of research education in undergraduate nursing programs and varying support from organisations for postgraduate research training for nurses.

The skills necessary to conduct EBP are easily identified and relate to competencies such as searching and retrieval of research literature, critical appraisal of research reports, and a level of skills in the design and conduct of epidemiological research. The skills and attitudes necessary to sustain a culture of inquiry are less easy to acquire and have been identified as having a professional pride and vision to build the evidence base for practice, being motivated and having the willingness, energy, enthusiasm, tenacity and ability to initiate change, being aware of their strengths and limitations, and having commitment to continuous learning (Bland & Ruffin 1992, McCormack & Garbett 2003, Scott et al 1999). Clinical academic positions that are joint appointments between a tertiary institution and the healthcare facility can play a major role in achieving change in this area by role modelling, promoting collaboration, supporting change agents and empirically demonstrating the value of EBP.

It may seem simple enough to provide resources for training programs and equipment needed to engage in EBP, but organisations have to do more. They have to provide an infrastructure that will not only sustain continual learning in EBP, but also support nurses in making changes based on the evidence. In most organisations clinical practice consumes all of nursing time with little time and space for development of that practice through questioning practice, reading research, and initiating and implementing innovations in practice. In short, in the contemporary healthcare environment there is insufficient time for nurses to engage in EBP.

The literature is clear that this is an organisational problem. The organisation needs to make time for nurses to develop their practice. However, organisational responsibility is only the first step. Time is a commodity in the clinical environment that is quickly consumed with patient care activities. For example, if an overlap time exists between shifts, this may well provide opportunity for nurses to plan new initiatives. However, what is likely to happen is that clinical care will encroach on this time. The work of patient care is unlimited and will expand to fill the time available. So, organisational responsibility is not the final answer. The challenge is for nurses to create their own practice development time.

After protected time for engaging in the EBP agenda is negotiated with nursing managers and made available through an organisational commitment to build time into existing work rosters, creation and protection of that time needs to come from the clinical staff. Teams must be facilitated to identify creative ways to ensure that negotiated practice development time is available. This requires a commitment from the whole team and a determination to own the problem and the solution. Nurse clinicians must collaborate with each other and take responsibility and control of their work environment to break down this time barrier.

Once the question of 'Why aren't nurses using research?' is attended to and barriers removed, organisations need to ask the questions, 'how' and 'what'. How can we shift the culture forward beyond exploration and towards integration of evidence with decision making, and what do nurses need to effect change in practice?

9.6.3 Support for autonomy and authority to change practice

As mentioned earlier in this chapter, autonomy has been defined as 'an individual's ability to independently carry out the responsibilities of the position without close supervision' and 'is closely linked to authority' (Blanchfield & Biordi 1996:43). In a concept analysis of the plethora of literature on autonomy Ballou (1998) found several emerging themes in the literature. Autonomy encompasses 'a self-governance system of principles, competence or capacity, decision-making, critical reflection, freedom, and self-control' (Ballou 1998:103). The literature demonstrates a strong association between autonomous decision making in clinical practice and job satisfaction, and perceived productivity in organisations where the nurse leader values education and professional development of all nurses (Scott et al 1999), which are key requisites in capacity building in EBP.

There is typically a lack of decision-making power by nurses related to patient management issues within the medically dominated health system hierarchy. Nursing clinical practice and medical practice are perceived as linked. However, nursing practice is more likely to be seen as dependent upon medical decision making. This perception, at times, has the effect of subsuming nurse decision making and autonomy over nursing practice to a task-oriented role under the direction of medicine. Healthcare is multidisciplinary and decisions made about patient care should reflect a true collaborative relationship between disciplines by relinquishing control over aspects of patient care management to those disciplines that have legitimate responsibility for those aspects of care. Relationships focused on optimising patient outcomes should replace relationships based on power.

Models of change that encourage clinicians to become evidence-based practitioners and strategies for assisting such change usually hinge on the organisation committing more resources, more time and more development. This enables the first three steps in the EBP process (i.e. formulate a question, find the evidence, appraise the evidence) to occur, but may not address the further steps of applying the evidence and evaluating the practice change. Literature abounds with strategies, models, plans and algorithms for implementing practice change and getting clinicians to buy into the change. This may be effective for nurse–nurse buy-in, but what about cross-disciplinary buy-in? Even practices that nurses have control over are influenced by other disciplines.

One example of this is wound care. Wound care has been a responsibility of nursing since Florence Nightingale. Nurses have managed wounds from pressure ulcers and vascular ulcers, to postoperative wounds and post-radiation therapy wounds to ostomy wounds. But why don't nurses have autonomous control over choice of wound management interventions? Even where there is strong evidence favouring a particular wound dressing intervention, the nurse clinician often, in many settings, perceives that they do not have the autonomy or authority to make the decision to evaluate a practice change. Nurses need to seize back the requisite autonomy and authority to make practice change decisions based on evidence and not be stopped by medical determination. Here is the place where a cultural or organisational change is needed. There is no magic bullet to changing an organisation to a culture of inquiry, but if the organisation is going to espouse to being an evidence-based organisation, all clinicians must be able to change their practice based on evidence, clinician judgment and patient values. Only then can the organisation truly be a culture of inquiry.

The EBP movement has both great potential and challenges for the development of the discipline of nursing. The potential of EBP is in two main areas:

1. It provides a scientific framework for building the practice knowledge base for nursing.
2. If harnessed, EBP can support clinical autonomy and advanced practice roles for nursing.

Clinical autonomy or decision-making influence over one's own practice comes with confidence in the knowledge base of that practice. Nursing has undergone a dramatic change in the past 20 years. In many countries the education of nurses at some, if not all, levels is conducted in the tertiary environment. As a consequence, nursing has developed and continues to develop a knowledge base through research and scholarly inquiry. Additionally, there is a vast amount of skill, knowledge and expertise in nursing practice. Nursing is lifesaving, it is therapeutic, it is caring, it is scientific and it is technological. And nursing is central to the operation of healthcare. This has become more evident in the recent and continuing global nursing shortage, which has resulted in a crisis in many healthcare systems. So, nursing has authority through its knowledge base, its expertise and its role in healthcare. The challenge for nurses in gaining authority to change practice is to continue to identify the domains of nursing practice and to systematically gather evidence to support best practice in these domains.

9.7 Examples of a culture of inquiry

Attempts are being made to develop cultures of inquiry in healthcare through several processes. Two examples, Magnet Hospitals, conceived and established in the United States, and Practice Development Units, established in the UK (although adopted and adapted in Australia), are described here to highlight similarities in the strategic aims, structure, processes and outcomes of each in establishing and maintaining a culture of inquiry in healthcare.

9.7.1 Magnet Hospitals

In 1982, the American Academy of Nursing (AAN) conducted its first 'Magnet' study to explore factors that affected recruitment and retention of professional nurses. The study found core organisational characteristics existed among 41 hospitals distinguished by high nurse satisfaction, low job turnover and low nurse vacancy rates (McClure et al 1983). The study found that an environment that supports nursing excellence was a key factor not only in attracting and retaining highly qualified nurses, but also in promoting positive patient care outcomes. Key characteristics of the original Magnet Hospitals included:

- a nurse executive was a formal member of the highest decision-making body in the organisation
- the nursing service was organised in a flat organisational structure
- decision making was decentralised to the unit level
- nurses on each unit were given responsibility for organising care and staffing appropriate to patient needs
- administrative structures supported nurses' decisions about care, and
- good communication existed between nurses and physicians (McClure et al 1983).

Today, the Magnet Hospital concept has been renewed and formalised in the Magnet Nursing Services Recognition Program™, which is administered by the American Nurses Credentialling Center (ANCC) and is based on the American Nurses Association's nursing quality indicators and standards of nursing practice.

The overall goal of the program is to recognise excellence in the provision of quality nursing care and acknowledge organisations that 'uphold the tradition within nursing of professional nursing practice' (ANCC 2003). The program also provides a medium for disseminating successful practices and strategies among nursing services (ANCC 2003). There has been a significant amount of research on the Magnet Hospital concept as a model of professional nursing practice since its inception demonstrating that Magnet Hospitals had better outcomes than non-Magnet Hospitals (McClure et al 1983, Scott et al 1999).

Subsequent research has highlighted other important characteristics that have an effect on recruitment and retention related to the hospital nurse leaders, such as: visibility and staff support; characteristics related to clinical nursing practice, such as autonomy and control within clinical practice, status within the organisation and collaboration across levels and disciplines; and characteristics related to the organisational culture, such as participative management and support of professional development (Kramer & Schmalenberg 2003a, 2003b, Scott et al 1999). More recent research suggests that Magnet Hospitals accredited under the ANCC program had even better outcomes than the original Magnet Hospitals (Scott et al 1999), and that there is an association between characteristics of professional nursing as demonstrated in Magnet Hospitals and the impact on patient outcomes, such as morbidity and mortality, and satisfaction with nursing care (Aiken et al 1994, Aiken et al 1996, Havens & Aiken 1999, Scott et al 1999). The ANCC Magnet Nursing Services Recognition Program™ 'offers an evidence-based model for nurse leaders interested in transforming the practice climate' (Stolzenberger 2003:522).

While the focus of Magnet Hospitals and the Magnet Hospital literature is on recruitment and retention of nurses, organisational characteristics aimed at improving recruitment and retention are key characteristics of organisations that support a culture of inquiry.

9.7.2 Practice Development Units

Another approach aimed at supporting a culture of inquiry has been suggested in contemporary literature, and is referred to as Practice Development. Practice Development Units have the potential to transcend the barriers to research utilisation in practice by strategically and systematically enhancing clinical effectiveness in patient health outcomes through best practice innovations, while stimulating a change in the culture and context of care (Manley & McCormack 2003).

Practice Development has its theoretical underpinning in critical social science. Critical social science is an attempt to understand in a rationally responsible manner the oppressive features of a society such that this understanding stimulates its audience to transform their society and thereby liberate themselves (Fay 1987). In other words, Practice Development, as a methodology, guides nurses away from the perception that they cannot make decisions and influence healthcare because of medical domination. The process takes them on a journey of discovery of the factors in their 'socio-professional' environment that inhibit and enable them to demonstrate their contribution to health outcomes to feeling empowered to participate in healthcare decisions. This is achieved by enabling them with the skills to interrogate and change from a practice based on traditions, rituals and myths to a practice based on evidence. Practice Development has been defined in contemporary literature as:

> *. . . a continuous process of increased effectiveness in person centred care through enabling of nurses to transform the culture and context of care . . . it is enabled and supported by facilitators committed to a systematic, rigorous and continuous process of emancipatory change (McCormack et al 1999:256).*

Nomenclature used in the literature to describe the concept of Practice Development is confusing. In the 1960s, there was the pioneering concept in the US of the 'Care, Core and Cure' model (Hall 1966). From this early concept, came the 1980s UK model of 'Nursing Development Units' initiated by Alan Pearson (Malby 1996, Salvage 1995). In Australia, the concept emerged as 'Clinical Development Units, Nursing' (Greenwood 1999). The concept continued to evolve in the UK to the 1990s model of 'Practice Development Units' (McCormack et al 1999). The change in nomenclature is accompanied by slight variations in the philosophy and focus of the concept of Practice Development. Regardless of the nomenclature used to label Practice Development, key components consistent with most descriptions of the concept include the following:
- responding to identified patients' needs
- improving services to patients
- utilisation of evidence to support practice
- improving the effectiveness of the service
- improving the professional's role, knowledge and/or skills, and
- empowering nurses to introduce change to improve practice (Greenwood 1999, McCormack & Garbett 2003, Pearson 1989, Salvage 1995, Unsworth 2000).

More recently, the importance of facilitation in ensuring the success of Practice Development has been advocated. A trained and experienced facilitator committed to enabling nurses to critically interrogate their practice using an evidence-based approach towards efficient and effective practice change through research is key (McCormack & Garbett 2003, McCormack et al 1999, Thompson et al 2001, Unsworth 2000). Clinically credible nurses within the practice environment, such as clinical nurse specialists, clinical educators and Practice Development nurses, provide the most effective route to enabling nurses to use research in practice (Thompson et al 2001). Practice Development methodology brings together, under the guidance of these trained and experienced facilitators, the simultaneous development of the nurse while improving outcomes for the patient using an EBP approach.

Although there is a plethora of literature on the nature and benefits of Practice Development (Greenwood 2000, Greenwood 1999, Kitson et al 1996, Manley & McCormack 2003, McCormack & Garbett 2003, McCormack et al 1999, Unsworth 2000), the term remains nebulous with clinicians (Clarke & Proctor 1999, Tolson 1999). In addition, there is little published literature systematically evaluating a Practice Development methodology in the Australian or international context (Draper 1996, Gerrish 2001). However, with its 'bottom-up' approach and theoretical underpinnings of critical social science theory, the central aim of Practice Development is to develop a culture of inquiry.

9.8 Conclusion

This chapter has explored the concepts of EBP and culture. We have also conceptualised what is meant by an 'evidence-based culture' and discussed in detail ways in which the organisation and the individual nurse can work together to achieve this 'culture of inquiry'. Without the requisite infrastructure, resources, support and incentives necessary to enable the development of practising evidence-based nursing and to enable the generation of nurse-initiated evidence for practice through the conduct of research, it will not be possible for organisations to sustain the transformation to a culture of inquiry.

9.9 Discussion questions

1. What are some of the characteristics of a culture of inquiry? Which of these characteristics are evident in your organisation?
2. What are some strategies for developing a culture of inquiry? What strategies could be used in your organisation?
3. Compare the Magnet Hospital concept with the Practice Development concept in relation to building a culture of inquiry. Consider which characteristics of each would suit your organisation's strategy for cultural change.

9.10 References

Aiken L H, Sloane D M, Lake E 1994 Lower Medicare mortality among a set of hospitals known for good nursing care. *Medical Care* 32:771–87.

Aiken L H, Sloane D M, Lake E 1996 Satisfaction with inpatient AIDS care: a national comparison of dedicated and scattered-bed units. *Medical Care* 35:948–62.

Aiken L H, Sloane D M, Lake E T et al 1999 Organization and outcomes of inpatient AIDS care. *Medical Care* 37:760–72.

American Nurses Credentialing Centre (ANCC) 2003 *ANCC Magnet Program—Recognizing excellence in nursing services.* Viewed 18 January 2003. Available at http://www.nursingworld.org/ancc/magnet.html.

Baggs J G, Schmitt M H, Mushlin A I et al 1999 Association between nurse–physician collaboration and patient outcomes in three intensive care units. *Critical Care Medicine* 27:1991–8.

Ballou K A 1998 A concept analysis of autonomy. *Journal of Professional Nursing* 14:102–10.

Bate P 1994 *Strategies for cultural change.* Butterworth-Heinemann, Oxford.

Blanchfield K C, Biordi D L 1996 Power in practice: a study of nursing authority and autonomy. *Nursing Administration Quarterly* Spring:42–9.

Bland C J, Ruffin M T 1992 Characteristics of a productive research environment: literature review. *Academic Medicine* 67:385–97.

Bryar R M, Closs S J, Baum G et al 2003 The Yorkshire BARRIERS project: diagnostic analysis of barriers to research utilisation. *International Journal of Nursing Studies* 40:73–84.

Clarke C, Proctor S 1999 Practice development: ambiguity in research and practice. *Journal of Advanced Nursing* 30(4):975–82.

Draper J 1996 Nursing development units: an opportunity for evaluation. *Journal of Advanced Nursing* 23:267–71.

Fay B 1987 *Critical social science*. Cornell University Press, Ithaca, New York.

Forbes A, Griffiths P 2002 Methodological strategies for the identification and synthesis of 'evidence' to support decision-making in relation to complex healthcare systems and practices. *Nursing Inquiry* 9:141–55.

Funk S G, Champagne M T, Wiese R A, Tornquist E M 1991 Barriers to using research findings in practice: the clinician's perspective. *Applied Nursing Research* 4:90–5.

Gerrish K 2001 A pluralistic evaluation of nursing/practice development units. *Journal of Clinical Nursing* 10(1):109–18.

Greenwood J 1999 Clinical development units (nursing): the Western Sydney approach. *Journal of Advanced Nursing* 29:674–9.

Greenwood J 2000 Clinical development units (nursing): issues surrounding their establishment and survival. *International Journal of Nursing Practice* 6:338–44.

Hall L E 1966 Another view of nursing care and quality, in M Straub & K Parker (eds), *Continuity of patient care: the role of nursing*. Catholic University of America Press, Washington, DC.

Havens D S 2001 Comparing nursing infrastructure and outcomes: ANCC magnet and nonmagnet CNEs report. *Nursing Economics* 19:258–66.

Havens D S, Aiken L H 1999 Shaping systems to promote desired outcomes: the Magnet Hospital model. *Journal of Nursing Administration* 29:14–20.

Havens D, Vasey J 2003 Measuring staff nurse decisional involvement. The decisional involvement scale. *Journal of Nursing Administration* 33:331–6.

Heater B S, Becker A M, Olson R K 1988 Nursing interventions and patient outcomes: a meta-analysis of studies. *Nursing Research* 37:303–7.

Hesselbein F 2002 The key to cultural transformation, in F Hesselbein & R Johnston (eds), *On leading change: a leader to leader guide*. Jossey-Bass, Indianapolis.

Holland C K 1993 An ethnographic study of nursing culture as an exploration for determining the existence of a system of ritual. *Journal of Advanced Nursing* 18:1461–70.

Kajermo K N, Nordstrom G, Krusebrant A, Bjorvell H 1998 Barriers to and facilitators of research utilization, as perceived by a group of registered nurses in Sweden. *Journal of Advanced Nursing* 27:798–807.

Kitson A, Ahmed L B, Harvey G et al 1996 From research to practice: one organizational model for promoting research-based practice. *Journal of Advanced Nursing* 23:430–40.

Kramer M, Schmalenberg C E 2003a Magnet Hospital nurses describe control over nursing practice. *Western Journal of Nursing Research* 25:434–52.

Kramer M, Schmalenberg C E 2003b Magnet Hospital staff nurses describe clinical autonomy. *Nursing Outlook* 51:13–19.

Malby R 1996 Nursing development units in the United Kingdom. *Advanced Practice Nursing Quarterly* 1:20–7.

Manley K, McCormack B 2003 Practice development: purpose, methodology, facilitation and evaluation. *Nursing in Critical Care* 8:22–9.

McClure M, Poulin M, Sovie M D 1983 *Magnet Hospitals: attraction and retention of professional nurses*. American Academy of Nurses, American Nurses Association, Kansas City.

McCormack B, Garbett R 2003 The characteristics, qualities and skills of practice developers. *Journal of Clinical Nursing* 12:317–25.

McCormack B, Manley K, Kitson A et al 1999 Towards practice development: a vision in reality or a reality without vision? *Journal of Nursing Management* 7:255–64.

Miller J R, Messenger S R 1978 Obstacles to applying nursing research findings. *American Journal of Nursing* 78:632–4.

O'Callaghan J 2001 Do rituals still rule over research evidence? *Australian Nursing Journal* 8:39–40.

Osborne S R, Gardner G 2004 Imperatives and strategies for developing an evidence-based practice in perioperative nursing. *ACORN Journal* 17(1):18–24.

Parahoo K 2001 Research utilization among medical and surgical nurses: a comparison of their self reports and perceptions of barriers and facilitators. *Journal of Nursing Management* 9:21–30.

Pearson A 1989 Therapeutic nursing: transforming models and theories in action. *Recent Advances in Nursing* 24:123–51.

Retsas A 2000 Barriers to using research evidence in nursing practice. *Journal of Advanced Nursing* 31:599–606.

Salvage J 1995 Greenhouses, flagships and umbrellas, in J Salvage & S G Wright (eds), *Nursing development units: a force for change*. Scutari Press, London.

Schein E H 1992 *Organizational culture and leadership,* 2nd edn. Jossey-Bass, San Francisco.

Scott J G, Sochalski J, Aiken L H 1999 Review of Magnet Hospital research: findings and implications for professional nursing practice. *Journal of Nursing Administration* 29:9–19.

Stolzenberger K M 2003 Beyond the Magnet award: the ANCC Magnet program as the framework for culture change. *Journal of Nursing Administration* 33:522–31.

Strange F 2002 The persistence of ritual in nursing practice. *Clinical Effectiveness in Nursing* 5:177–83.

Thompson C, McCaughan D, Cullum N et al 2001 The accessibility of research-based knowledge for nurses in United Kingdom acute care settings. *Journal of Advanced Nursing* 36:11–22.

Tolson D 1999 Practice innovation: a methodological maze. *Journal of Advanced Nursing* 30(2):381–90.

Tranmer J E, Coulson K, Holtom D et al 1998 The emergence of a culture that promotes evidence based clinical decision making within an acute care setting. *Canadian Journal of Nursing Administration* 11:36–58.

Unsworth J 2000 Practice development: a concept analysis. *Journal of Nursing Management* 8:317–26.

Webb S S, Price S A, Van Ess Coeling H 1996 Valuing authority/responsibility relationships: the essence of professional practice. *Journal of Nursing Administration* 26:28–33.

Winslow E H 1998 Questioning the chains of habit. *The Journal of Cardiovascular Nursing* 12:94–108.

chapter 10

Undertaking a clinical audit

Sally Borbasi, Debra Jackson and Craig Lockwood

10.1 Learning objectives

After reading this chapter, you should be able to:

1. *define what is meant by the term 'clinical audit'*
2. *understand how clinical audit fits within the framework of quality improvement*
3. *discuss the differences and similarities between audit and research*
4. *explain why clinical audits are useful, and*
5. *describe the major steps in the clinical audit process.*

10.2 Introduction

Evidence-based healthcare has made huge inroads over the last few years. There have been a number of bodies formed to produce and disseminate best evidence, and as a result a massive discourse has grown around the topic. Resources for quick access to information on best practice are plentiful and readily available to both practitioners and consumers. Yet, despite this mass of activity and expenditure in producing evidence it has become clear that putting it into practice has been less successful. Indeed uptake of evidence remains one of the key challenges facing nurses internationally (Borbasi et al 2004). The literature is full of interventions and ideas to help enhance the uptake of evidence into clinical practice. However, Thompson and Learmonth (2002:236) suggest that interventions such as didactic study days, and passively disseminated clinical guidelines and protocols, have 'little or no effect on practice'.

One tool that has been effective in advancing evidence-based practice (EBP) is the clinical audit. The clinical audit has been situated primarily in the final (fifth) phase of the evidence-based cycle and concerns evaluation (i.e. it follows after the first four phases of: formulating a clinical question; locating the evidence; critically appraising the evidence; and then applying the evidence to bring about change). Evaluation determines the effect of an intervention on clinical practice/patients. Indeed, there is 'no point trying to evidence base your practice if you have no commitment to evaluate the outcomes of your care' (ACEBCP 2003:100). Thus, clinical audit is a tool to evaluate care (Mason 2002) and with evaluation the EBP cycle begins again. Indeed, as Mason (2002:295) points out, any audit should be completed by 'follow-up audits'.

This chapter introduces the concept of clinical audit as a tool that is increasingly being used in clinical environments under the aegis of EBP and quality improvement. The reader is provided with an overview of clinical audit as a way to develop knowledge and enhance clinical practice, including exploration of the usefulness of audit and of how to actually conduct one.

10.3 What is a clinical audit?

Clinical audit is a tool used by healthcare professionals to examine their practice and compare the outcomes either with quality standards, clinical guidelines or best practice evidence. In effect, clinical audit is a quality improvement process that aims to identify how to improve clinical practice, or to demonstrate that best practice standards are being met through current methods of care provision (Kinn 1995).

The primary goals of clinical audit are to improve patient care, and related outcomes, and to promote the implementation of best practice evidence. The process used to conduct an audit can vary, but tends to be based on a series of related activities incorporating a varied number of steps— depending on the complexity of the topic chosen (commonly a four- or five-step process is described). Best practice or other standards are introduced to the practice setting, current practice is then audited and compared with best practice standards, outcomes are measured, and practice is changed if the audit results indicate a need for change. This process is repeated over time to ensure any changes to practice are maintained, and that patient outcomes continue to improve. As the ideal method of audit is to repeat it over time, audit has been described as a cyclical process that may be continuously, or intermittently, applied. A more formal definition of clinical audit suggests it is a:

> . . . quality improvement process that seeks to improve patient care and outcomes through systematic review of care against explicit criteria and the implementation of change. Aspects of the structure, processes and outcomes of care are selected and systematically evaluated against explicit criteria. Where indicated, changes are implemented at an individual, team or service level and further monitoring is used to confirm improvement in health-care delivery (NICE 2004).

Clinical audit then is a quality improvement and a change process based on the evaluation of current practice. Morrell and Harvey (1999:10) describe four main stages of clinical audit. The process begins by clearly defining best practice (stage 1); once this is established there is a move to implement best practice (stage 2), so bringing about change. This is followed by monitoring (stage 3) and comparing actual practice and outcomes against best practice standards (stage 4). Findings from this stage should lead to action to improve practice.

The National Institute for Clinical Excellence (NICE) (2002:101–4) presents principles for best practice in clinical audit that incorporate an additional fifth stage. In addition to the steps described by Morrell and Harvey (1999),

149

NICE (2002) include a stage for sustaining the improvements resulting from the practice change component of audit. The emphasis on sustainable change is valid and important given the varying effectiveness of ensuring worthwhile, long-term practice change in the care of patients (Walshe & Spurgeon 1997). The steps described by NICE involve preparing for audit, selecting criteria, measuring the level of performance, making improvements and sustaining improvement. These steps provide a framework rather than actual instructions for how to conduct an audit; hence a detailed example is provided later in this chapter.

Shakib (2003) describes audit as a tool for determining the current state of a situation and, once results are determined, for bringing about change to best practice. Morrell and Harvey (1999) on the other hand refer to audit as a tool used to monitor and evaluate best practice after best practice has been implemented. Their model involves the development and implementation of best practice standards into care that is then followed up by audit.

Either way, it can be seen that audit is really all about improving patient care. It is never static; both of the models described above include a need for continual reaudit. Audit is also a useful tool to establish a baseline for later comparison when considering change in practice. Baseline audits assist in identifying and prioritising areas of guideline-related practice that require change (Perry 2002:261).

After the change has been implemented repeat audits serve to evaluate whether there have been any gains from it. Perry (2002:261) points out that audit may be a way of 'selling' change, as it offers promise of evaluation, which is something clinicians often complain is not forthcoming. However, Thompson and Learmonth (2002:230) warn that on its own clinical audit is probably not a sufficient mechanism for bringing about sustained change and that a number of multifaceted strategies for change should be put in place. These may include electronic or paper-based reminders and educational programs (Thompson & Learmonth 2002: 236).

Though many clinical audits are conducted locally, Mason (2002) advocates national audits over and above local audit projects, which he claims, for a variety of reasons, tend not to produce better health outcomes. He states, 'the future of clinical audit, as a major agent of change, lies with nationally organised projects associated with national priorities' (Mason 2002:296). UK national audits have included the Myocardial Infarction National Audit Project and the National Sentinel Audit for Stroke, both of which have utilised all the very latest in information technology, rapid feedback to stakeholders and reaudit. Other national clinical audits undertaken in the UK include the management of elderly people who have fallen, the management of violence in mental health settings, the management of patients with venous leg ulcers and audit of the use of caesarean section (NICE 2002:94).

10.4 How does a clinical audit relate to the quality improvement movement?

In an effort to improve the quality of clinical practice over the last few years a number of initiatives have emerged, the names of which have changed as 'new groups of management gurus' have refashioned and reshaped former ideas (Mason 2002:294). Thus, terminology surrounding the notion of providing best care is dynamic. For example, until recently, clinical effectiveness has been popular, but now the wider concept of clinical governance has come into vogue. In the UK, Morell and Harvey (1999:10) see clinical audit as part of clinical effectiveness and quality improvement, whereas Mason (2002) states clinical audit has become an integral component of the clinical governance processes within the National Health Service (NHS). Both are correct. Clinical governance is the framework through which clinical effectiveness takes place, and is intended as an accountability model focused on creating environments that seek to safeguard high standards of care and continuously improve them (Gaston 2003).

Clinical effectiveness has been defined as:

> . . . applying the best available knowledge, derived from research,
> clinical expertise and patient preferences, to achieve optimum
> processes and outcomes of care for patients (Royal College of
> Nursing 1996, cited in Morell & Harvey 1999:11).

Clinical audit is regarded as an integral part of any clinical effectiveness program (Morrell & Harvey 1999:156), whereas clinical governance is seen as:

> . . . a system through which . . . organisations are accountable
> for continuously improving the quality of their services and
> safeguarding high standards of care by creating an environment
> in which excellence in clinical care will flourish
> (Scally & Donaldson 1998:61).

It divides quality into four aspects:
1. professional performance (technical quality)
2. resource use (efficiency)
3. risk management (the risk of injury or illness associated with the service provided), and
4. patients' satisfaction with the service provided (WHO 1983, cited in Scally & Donaldson 1998:61).

NICE in the UK believe 'clinical audit is at the heart of clinical governance' (NICE 2002:vi). NICE have produced a book called *Principles for best practice in clinical audit*, which can be downloaded free from the NICE website. The book addresses the five stages of clinical audit: preparation; selecting criteria; measuring performance; making improvements; and sustaining that improvement.

Another useful resource is a computer package called Auditmaker designed by Sepehr Shakib through the Australian Centre for Evidence Based Clinical Practice (ACEBCP). This package is available free from the ACEBCP website following initial registration. It can be used to guide you through the first steps of designing an audit, in determining the factors and outcomes that require analysis and then to provide easily customised data-entry forms and simple reports to summarise the data. The designers describe it as 'user-friendly', having drop-down lists, help buttons and in-built comorbidities and outcomes of common interest (Shakib 2003:1). The Auditmaker tool provides a generic instrument for performing an audit in addition to providing opportunity for differing groups of clinicians from across institutions or practice settings to use the same data-collection tool in order to benchmark practice (Shakib 2003:1). The Auditmaker package is used to illustrate aspects of audit in this chapter and selected elements of a real-live audit are drawn from an example provided by the Joanna Briggs Institute.

As described in Chapter 1, the National Institute of Clinical Studies (NICS) was established by the Australian Federal Government in 2000, and commenced operations in 2001. The primary purpose of the NICS is to champion continuous improvement in the quality and delivery of clinical practice to the Australian community. The methods by which this is to be achieved are based on partnership with consumers, health professionals and organisations, researchers and governments. In collaboration with these groups, NICS seeks to close the gaps between evidence and clinical practice, in those areas that will effect significant change for the Australian community by providing practitioners and health organisations with systems that will assist them to improve the health outcomes of those within their care.

The methods utilised in NICS projects vary according to the topic in question, although the focus across all projects is implementation of evidence in practice. Evaluations of projects and programs initiated by NICS reflect similarity to audit programs in that there are distinct barriers and facilitators to change. The challenge to address these in context-specific ways is being addressed by NICS through the development of reference groups with the role of establishing a coordinated national approach to implementation. The parallels with optimal audit program design include use of multidisciplinary approaches, use of broad-based programs to target key clinical problems identified via research, and then using multiple methods to close the gaps between evidence and practice. Details of some of the work of NICS were presented in Appendix 1.1 in Chapter 1.

10.5 What do clinical audits measure?

The UK-based NICE states that 'clinical audits monitor the use of particular interventions, or the care received by patients, against agreed standards'. Effectiveness is the degree to which an intervention does what it is meant to do in normal circumstances (Thomas 1999). In assessing effectiveness, evidence is needed to determine if intended outcomes were achieved. The clinical audit process is a way of ascertaining the achievement or failure of intended outcomes. It allows the identification of departure from 'best practices so that they can be examined in order to understand and act upon the causes' (NICE at www.nice.org.uk/article.asp?a=953).

Thomas (1999:41) differentiates clinical audit from medical audit by defining the former as being concerned with the 'total package of care offered to patients', rather than focusing only on the medical care. The clinical audit focuses on nursing care, service provision and management, as well as physical and environmental issues (Thomas 1999). This positions the clinical audit as an essentially multidisciplinary activity, which is in keeping with the fact that the provision of health services is also a multidisciplinary activity (Closs & Cheater 1996).

10.6 Audit or research?

Nurses have been evaluating their work for years but have not actually called that process audit (Kinn 1995). In nursing circles, what began as medical audits have now become clinical audits (Mason 2002), and clinical audits have come to be viewed as an important aspect of professional accountability

(NICE 2002:8). There is some contention over whether or not clinical audits are research and therefore require approval from an institutional ethics committee (IEC). Scott (2000) is convinced clinical audit is research, whereas CRAG (the Clinical Resource and Audit Group) in Scotland categorically takes the view that because research is about establishing new knowledge, audit is not research (cited Morrell & Harvey 1999:3).

Balogh (1996) also points out that research is concerned with extending knowledge, whereas audits are concerned with making sure that best current knowledge is being applied in practice and promoting positive practice change. However, Balogh (1996) acknowledges the similarities between audit and research, in that they both engage in a process of inquiry, and both employ similar strategies for gathering and analysing information (similarly Mead & Moseley 1996). Closs and Cheater (1996) highlight further differences in the two processes in that audit is theorised as a repeating, circular process, whereas with some exceptions, research is more often conceptualised as linear in nature. Furthermore, whereas much research aims to be generalisable, audits are carried out in local environments, and therefore reflect practices in a particular setting (Balogh 1996). The nature of the clinical audit can be likened to the action research cycle, which also focuses on local solutions to local problems and engages in a process of data collection to facilitate practice change.

No matter where one sits in the debate, it is clear that undertaking a clinical audit can contribute to research by drawing attention to areas requiring further research, as well as raising new researchable areas (Balogh 1996). Audit is a mechanism by which the gap between research and practice can be closed by comparing the two, identifying any inconsistencies, and guiding the development of methods to improve practice in the light of research findings. Despite the controversy, it is clear that clinical audits do raise ethical issues (e.g. use of patient records to gather information). Therefore, they should adhere to the same ethical principles common to any sphere of clinical practice, investigation or research, and require approval from an institutional body specifically set up to assess such proposals, such as an IEC (Morrell & Harvey 1999:105, NICE 2002).

10.7 Why are clinical audits useful in practice development?

There are a number of advantages to clinical audit. Ideally the audit should be a routine part of care (Closs & Cheater 1996) and so produce a constant spiral of intervention–monitoring–review of clinical care. Kinn (1995:36) points out that raising standards of care can only benefit patient outcomes and that the provision of care will be more efficient, which should enhance the job satisfaction of staff. Audit is seen to be educational and a useful tool for fostering interdisciplinary teamwork and communication. Morrell and Harvey (1999:158) state that clinical audit provides an avenue for reflection on work by healthcare workers, which, in turn, facilitates the development of their practice, knowledge and attitudes. The development of practice and the development of practitioners are regarded as inextricably linked (Morrell et al 1995, cited in Morrell & Harvey 1999:158).

NICE point out that effective clinical audit is important for a range of stakeholders, including health professionals, health service managers, patients and the public. They explain that audits:

- support health professionals in ensuring their patients receive the best possible care
- inform health service managers of the need for organisational change, or new investment to support health professionals in their practice
- assist in ensuring that patients are given the best possible care, and
- provide the public with confidence in the quality of the service as a whole (NICE at www.nice.org.uk/article.asp?a=953).

10.8 The process of undertaking a clinical audit

Considerations in setting up an audit include whether it will use a top-down or bottom-up approach, the time available, the need for extra resources and whether the audit problem is in an area where any changes will have 'a real effect on the immediate working environment' (Kinn 1995:36).

Morrell and Harvey (1999) restate that the fundamental principles underpinning a clinical audit include that it should:
- be professionally led
- be seen as an educational process
- form a part of routine clinical practice
- be based on the setting of standards
- generate results that can be used to improve outcome of quality care
- involve management in both the process and outcome of audit
- be confidential at the individual patient/clinician level, and
- be informed by the views of patients/clients (Department of Health UK 1993, cited in Morrell & Harvey 1999:2–3).

In conducting a clinical audit there are a number of factors to consider. Shakib (2003:17) calls these 'audit fundamentals', and while some may not be compulsory they are important because they promote a carefully thought out and systematic approach to the task. Prudent planning in the early stages makes for increased efficiency throughout the process.

Any clinical audit needs a written (or computer-generated) proposal. This information is used to apply for either ethical approval or perhaps to an audit committee, if that is the institution's policy. The proposal should include a title and a location for the audit (e.g. 'prospective audit of intravenous cannulations in Wards 5Y and 5Z'). The names of all the people who will be significantly involved in conducting the audit are included. These staff are usually those who have constructed the aims and objectives behind the audit and who have a good understanding of the issues involved (Shakib 2003). It is essential the audit have 'a clear purpose and clear aims' (Shakib 2003:19), and so justification for its conduct is unmistakable. The specific outcomes of the project and the endpoints to be measured need to be spelt out, and consideration given to any factors that might influence the outcomes of interest. For example, it would be important to know how long cannulas were routinely left in place in Ward 5Y as opposed to Ward 5Z, and who was responsible for replacing the cannulas in each ward.

Inclusion criteria are the factors defining the population you want to study. These need to be carefully identified (Shakib 2003:21). For example, you may want to include only those patients who have cannulas inserted on the ward—not those who received one in the Emergency Department or who have been transferred from another ward/hospital. Exclusion criteria are those factors you are not interested in exploring (e.g. you may only want to look at peripheral cannulas, not central lines).

Shakib (2003:21) suggests there needs to be some thought given to what the team thinks the audit will find. In this way the outcomes and the factors that impact on the outcomes can be selected 'in such a way as to highlight the aspects of the results that you are interested in' (Shakib 2003:21). He strongly reinforces the view of there being absolutely no point in conducting an audit unless there is firm commitment to acting on the results. Some pre-empting of what the audit may show allows the team to start thinking about inter-vention strategies and reauditing. This means the team may opt to collect slightly different data in order to make the intervention/s and reauditing easier (Shakib 2003:21).

The next section of the proposal contains reference to the methods you are going to use to collect your data. Shakib (2003) urges rigour in data collection. Morrell and Harvey (1999:49) refer to the importance of good measurement. As there is a real probability the audit will demonstrate a need to change prac-tice, the results must be believable and data-collection and analysis processes open to scrutiny. When 'unsavoury' audit data are presented, staff tend to mount their defences and any weaknesses in the audit process are quickly spotted (Morrell & Harvey 1999:22) rendering results (and thus the need to change practice/s) much less convincing. It is important to remember that an overemphasis on rigour 'risks alienating the very people likely to benefit from involvement in clinical audit' (Morrell & Harvey 1999:49), and so the relational aspects to audit need to be borne in mind. Indeed Morrell and Harvey (1999:9) are quick to stress a collaborative multiprofessional approach to audit and the benefits of the process to team building.

The sources of audit data can include, for example, questionnaires, inter-views, direct observation, as well as pre-existing sources such as medical records, patient notes and discharge data.

Several aspects of the sampling procedure need to be determined, not least of which are how many patients are required and whether they will be randomly selected and in within what time frame. Other considerations include:
- Who will collect the data?
- Will it be retrospectively or prospectively collected?
- Will consent be required?
- How will the data be recorded?
- How will it be analysed?
- What unanticipated hiccups might there be along the way (e.g. non-compliant staff)? (For greater depth see, for example, Shakib 2003, NICE 2002, Morrell & Harvey 1999.)

After the data are collected they need to be analysed and a summary of the findings written up and presented to the clinical audit group for interpreta-tion. The audit summary needs to provide constructive feedback, bearing in mind areas of both high and low achievement (Morrell & Harvey 1999:69). This is so that the group can look at ways to extrapolate success into areas requiring improvement. In this way clinical audit becomes less threatening to staff and does not just focus on negative aspects (Morrell & Harvey 1999:70).

The next step in the audit cycle is often the most problematic and involves planning for improvement or bringing about change. This is where a know-ledge of change theory becomes important. There are many texts devoted entirely to strategies/theories to bring about change; they make essential reading for clinicians wanting to implement best practice. After change has been implemented, there needs to be regular reaudit and review (usually in six-monthly or annual cycles); a report is often required and presentation of the project to a steering group or other interested parties. Publication to disseminate certain information regarding your audit is also a possibility. It is also a good idea for the audit team to come together for some reflection on how the audit went and what might be done differently the next time (Morrell & Harvey 1999:84).

Organisational support for clinical auditing is paramount to its success and is increasingly being provided through the establishment of clinical governance suites in many Australian healthcare facilities. The most commonly cited barrier to successful audit is the failure of an organisation to provide staff with the necessary protected time to carry out the work (NICE 2002:153). In addition, institutions need to recognise that audits require adequate funding and that changes to practice resulting from audits can actually increase costs especially in the first instance (NICE 2002:154). Yet, sustaining the improvements made to patient care through audit is essential to the success of clinical governance. Monitoring and evaluating change is advocated through reaudit and review. Maintaining and reinforcing change over time includes the need for:

- reinforcing or motivating factors to be built in by management to support the continual cycle of quality improvement
- integration of audit into the organisation's wider quality improvement systems, and
- strong leadership (NICE 2002:62).

10.9 Case study: example of an audit

In the following sections, the process of conducting a clinical audit is described drawing, by way of example, from an audit that has actually been completed. The framework used is detailed and can be used or adapted as required. This outline can also be used to form the basis of an audit protocol, which is a highly recommended component of the audit process. The benefits of writing an audit protocol are that it clarifies exactly the methods and structure of the audit, and it enhances communication and collaboration with key stakeholders.

This section utilises the following framework:

- topic selection
- question development and objectives
- identifying best practice
- audit indicator development
- implementing the standard/s (best practice)
- method
- sampling/data collection
- evaluation
- feedback, and
- reauditing.

10.9.1 Topic selection

When selecting an audit topic, priority should be given to selection of topics in areas where significant improvements to clinical care can be made—achieving the best outcome for your efforts should be kept in mind. There should be practical ways to make improvements or changes to the area of care if the clinical audit is going to be of any benefit. As clinical audit aims to compare current practice with an accepted standard, it is useful to identify high-quality standards (such as the Joanna Briggs Institute *Best Practice* information sheets) and/or develop an audit topic that can be used to compare practice with research evidence, such as systematic reviews or randomised controlled trials.

Factors to consider when thinking about a topic for clinical audit include:
- Do stakeholders have identified concerns with the issue (e.g. complaints)?
- Is there a wide variation in current practice for no obvious beneficial reason?
- Is it an area of high patient risk (e.g. high level of morbidity and/or mortality)?
- Is it an area of high volume (e.g. is it something that is done frequently)?
- Is it an area of high cost (e.g. will you be able to reduce or justify the cost)?
- Is there access to the necessary resources to complete the audit (e.g. time, information, staff) (Burnett & Winyard 1998, Morrell & Harvey 1999)?

In the audit that follows (Table 10.1), the topic selected was postoperative management of split thickness skin graft donor sites. The care of these wounds was principally a nursing responsibility; thus if practice change was found to be required, the responsibility was clearly within the nursing domain rather than across professional boundaries. Also, donor sites were managed on a single ward, making the audit simple to complete, and any required changes easier to negotiate than would have been the case if the audit included multiple wards.

10.9.2 Question development and objectives

After a topic or practice area has been chosen, it helps to clarify your ideas into a question that others can clearly link to the audit process—the more specific the better. The topic of donor sites was too general to investigate; hence a specific question was developed from the identified problem.
- *Identified problem.* Patients with split skin donor site graft dressings were having frequent dressing changes. The dressing changes were made using numerous product types with the aim of reinforcing or replacing the perioperative dressing when strikethrough occurred.
- *Specific question.* 'Is current practice in the management of split thickness skin graft donor site dressings based on the best available evidence?'

After the question had been established, objectives are developed to maintain the focus of activity. Objectives are outcome statements that indicate the quality target for the audit. Objectives should be expressed as outcomes statements such as: 'to ensure that practice related to indwelling urethral catheter care reduces the risk of infection'.

The primary objective of the audit described in Table 10.1 was to ensure donor site dressing management was congruent with the best available evidence. The question and objective clearly indicate the focus of the audit.

10.9.3 Identifying best practice

After the topic for auditing has been clearly stated, a guideline (preferably evidence-based) should be identified which establishes what best practice is and how it is to be achieved. The guideline can then be used to develop audit indicators. Accessing pre-established guidelines, systematic reviews, individual research trials and clinical databases to find evidence of best practice is the quickest and potentially most reliable method of identifying guidelines from which to develop measurable audit indicators (Morrell & Harvey 1996).

Audit indicators should be based on evidence that they are clinically effective and relevant, and are the basic measure against which practice is compared. *They concisely describe the quality of care to be achieved in definable and measurable terms.* Audit indicators based on best practice evidence provide the most reliable framework for audit activity. In the example in Table 10.1, the audit indicators are based on specific clinical guidelines from a *Best Practice* information sheet developed by the Joanna Briggs Institute (JBI). This demonstrates the link between best evidence, and audit indicator development.

In developing or adapting care standards, it is important that the resulting care standards are:
- relevant to local needs, including the needs of patients, staff, managers, the facility and consumers
- based on clear evidence
- reliable (able to be applied in the same way by different staff), and
- valid (the intended outcome will be achieved if the standard is adhered to) (Burnett & Winyard 1998).

The clinical guideline chosen for the audit topic will be used retrospectively during the clinical audit to assess the quality of the practice that occurred. To use clinical guidelines to assess practice they need to be developed into quantitative criteria, or 'indicators'. Indicators are defined as:

> *Quantitative statements that are used to measure quality of care.*
> *Indicators always include a percentage, ratio or other quantitative*
> *way of saying how many patients the expected care should be*
> *provided for (NCCA 1997).*

10.9.4 Audit indicator development

Indicators must be measurable, observable, relating to only one specific area of practice and be focused on the goal of achieving the best outcome for patients. This will ensure there is a clear means of evaluating whether day-to-day practice is meeting the care standards (Garland & Corfield 1999, Kinn 1995).

Look closely at each audit indicator and decide how data will be collected to determine whether the standard has been met. It is helpful to identify criteria that need to be met to achieve the standard in terms of the structure, process and outcome framework. This allows the audit to expand beyond examining outcomes, by including aspects of resource requirements, and practical activities that may impact on the outcomes; hence it is a more encompassing approach.

Structure criteria are the resources, or what is needed to implement the standard. These may include availability of staff, specific equipment or resources such as time required.

A *process criterion* refers to what needs to be done to implement the care standard—the actions to take and the decisions to make. The process will include aspects such as assessment, evaluation, referral, documentation and specific practical interventions. Examples of process criteria include assessment scales or tools, or care processes to enhance or correct skill and knowledge deficits.

Outcome criteria are the anticipated results of the intervention—what you are expecting to achieve through implementing the care standard. They should contain statements that are measurable, such as percentages or ratios (Morrell & Harvey 1996, Morrell & Harvey 1999, Kinn 1995).

10.9.5 Implementing the standard/s (best practice)

After the care standard and audit indicators have been developed, the expected standard of care needs to be distributed to all stakeholders and implemented. Practitioners, managers and patients should know the expected outcomes of interventions that are initiated and how they can most effectively achieve the outcomes. Sharing the standards of best practice allows those who will be affected by them to give some input or feedback to the audit team. For effective implementation of any change in practice it is important that staff members feel a 'sense of ownership'. Exchanging information and being open to feedback from colleagues will raise awareness of your audit activity, encourage communication and improve the adoption rate of new practice guidelines.

Depending on the complexity of the standard or the size of the organisation you are working in, you may need to allow more or less time between implementation of the standard/s and the clinical audit. A basic rule of thumb is to allow enough time for implementation, without allowing so much time that the project loses momentum. In the example in Table 10.1, the *Best Practice* standards had been circulated months prior to the audit, and all staff had been given the opportunity to read and gain familiarity with the recommendations for practice.

10.9.6 Method

Participation in audit is generally voluntary. It is common practice to develop an audit protocol, which is used to invite participation, and to seek permission from the appropriate people within your organisation. After approval has been obtained, identify and discuss the audit with key stakeholders (clinician groups, and/or those with a vested interest in the methods or outcomes of the audit) to gather support for the project. In the example in Table 10.1, the audit was conducted in a tertiary teaching hospital; hence permission was sought from the director of nursing for the service unit involved, and once obtained, a meeting was set up with the clinical nurse consultant and clinicians to explain the audit, and to obtain their support.

Data collection was by examination of clinical documentation, including medical records and hospital procedure manuals. The audit was conducted over four weeks, and surveyed all patients who underwent procedures that involved a split thickness skin graft donor site. Twenty patients were identified during the survey period with either a single ($n = 15$) or two or more ($n = 5$) donor sites.

10.9.7 Sampling/data collection

The key issue in audit sampling is to identify the sample size you require so that you can demonstrate a need for change in practice, or that practice is based on the best available evidence. For example, if the first 10 cases audited are found to be below best practice standards, clearly a problem exists that needs to be addressed—regardless of what the other cases show.

Identify the population—ask whether the entire population can or should be audited (e.g. time and financial constraints may dictate choosing a sample). The sample size should be large enough to give an overall representation of the practice within your facility/area. Be pragmatic! Collecting huge volumes of data looks impressive, but may not be necessary, so collect only what you need in order to address your audit indicators.

Data-collection tools such as checklists or questionnaires can be designed specifically for the audit or can be adapted from pre-existing collection tools (such as the example in Table 10.1). When collecting and recording the data, be considerate of basic research principles such as ethical considerations and confidentiality. Collecting data is the most visible part of the audit process.

In the example, audit data was collected by short answer/closed ended questionnaire. The findings of the questions were compiled into the audit outline as percentages of expected and achieved outcomes. The results showed that the primary dressings applied in the perioperative setting were either *Duoderm* or *Kaltostat*, both of which are moist wound-healing products. Of the identified donor sites, 15 required further reinforcement or change of dressing, and two did not require any additional intervention. A total of 114 extra items were used, including combines, crepe bandages, *Duoderm*, *Hyparfix* and *Chux*.

The reasons for reinforcement or replacement of dressings were as follows:
- leakage of exudates from the primary dressing
- primary dressing removed by patient
- *Kaltostat* changed to *Duoderm* to decrease risk of adherence to the wound bed, and
- pseudomonas infection present in the wound.

10.9.8 Evaluation

Evaluating data involves comparing the findings on day-to-day practice to the care standards outlining expected practice. To do this, actual findings are compared to the indicators that were developed during the first stage of audit. Where the standards of practice have not been met, a thorough audit will look at *why* best practice has not occurred. Understanding why the day-to-day practice that was observed did not meet the care standards is important for the next stage of audit—developing an action plan. Using multiple data-collection techniques that look at the structures, processes and outcomes will help establish the cause of the problem. Your analysis might find that care practices did meet the standards that were defined from best evidence and that the outcomes of care were being achieved in the most effective manner. It is important to feed this finding back to the facility stakeholders.

In evaluating the audit data in the example, current practice was not found to be consistent with best practice. While the primary dressings were moist wound-healing products, the number of additional products being used, and the reports of strikethrough as a cause of dressing changes/reinforcement, suggest perioperative dressing selection and ward-based protocols could be improved to increase the use of primary dressings with additional moisture-bearing capacities, and to increase the use of additional reinforcing rather than replacement. The range of additional dressing products being applied could also be reduced, promoting greater consistency in patient care delivery, and potentially reducing costs.

10.9.9 Feedback

There is a range of views on what to do once you have collected the audit data, with some sources suggesting you should evaluate the data and return to the key stakeholders with that information for them to discuss, and potentially develop further action frameworks (Morrell & Harvey 1999). However, this approach relies on the use of an audit group who will assist in the audit process, and in establishing an action plan once the data has been collected and evaluated. These resources are not always available; hence it is useful to make a list of potential methods for communicating the audit results where they will be most effective. Consider avenues of personal one-to-one communication, in addition to group presentations, and written communication through available resources.

The value of feedback of audit results is that it enhances a sense of ownership, people get to see the effects of their practice, and although potentially a threatening scenario, it can be highly motivating. Feedback should be carefully considered and structured to gain the most benefit (i.e. increase the likelihood that practice change will continue and be sustained). Poorly constructed feedback (e.g. criticism that is not constructive or that is not well presented) may undo previous good work at stimulating practice improvement.

10.9.10 Reauditing

The first issue to consider is whether and with what frequency the topic warrants reauditing. If reauditing would not be useful, it is likely the initial audit was not useful either; however, the frequency with which to reaudit is sometimes less easy to establish. Some aspects of practice require continuous audit. These include quality and safety standards, incident monitoring and key performance indicator outcomes.

The minimum duration between audit and reaudit should be the time frame required for all the initial indicators to be implemented. The time frame should also include consideration of staff workloads, other concurrent activities, key stakeholder interest and momentum.

A rule of thumb is to allow six months between audits of topics that do not require continuous monitoring. However, if the audit criteria were developed from evidence or guidelines that are updated regularly, the timing of the updates, particularly if there is a clinically significant change in the update, can be used as a guide. A follow-up audit will then provide a useful data set that identifies where practice change has been achieved, and those areas that require further work—thus indicating the sustainability of changes that have been effected.

Table 10.1 Example clinical audit

Facility/ward: _____ **Clinical auditing program:** _____

Audit topic: *Split thickness skin graft donor sites: post-harvest management* **Date:** _____

Related standards: JBI *Best Practice* information sheet 6(2) 2002

Audit objectives: *To measure the care interventions patients receive in relation to the post-harvest management of split thickness skin graft donor sites*

Rationale: *Clinical experience suggests care is varied, and that patients were experiencing ongoing problems with wound leakage and use of multiple dressing changes*

Audit team: *Clinicians and data collectors directly involved in the audit process*

Clinical guideline	Audit indicator
1. The primary dressing is a moist wound-healing product	1. ___100___ % of dressing products applied will be moist wound-healing products
2. The size and type of primary dressing applied is appropriate for the anticipated volume of exudate	2. ___100___ % of dressing selections will be based on anticipated volumes of exudate
3. The primary dressing is left intact and reinforced if required for the first 24–48 hours postoperatively	3. ___100___ % of primary dressings and reinforcement will be left intact for 24–48 hours postoperatively

Reference: JBI Best Practice *information sheet 6(2) 2002.*

Audit indicators

1. 100% of dressing products applied will be moist wound-healing products

Structure	Process	Outcome
S1 Theatre guidelines indicate moist wound-healing products should be used	P1 Moist wound-healing products are available in the perioperative setting	O1 Moist wound-healing products are applied as the primary dressing

2. 100% of dressing selections will be based on anticipated volumes of exudate

Structure	Process	Outcome
S2 Theatre guidelines recommend dressing selection based on anticipated moisture-absorbing requirements of the primary dressing	P2 Estimated wound fluid loss is evaluated as part of the dressing selection criteria	O2 Primary dressing applied is of appropriate size and moisture-bearing capacity for the donor site

3. 100% of primary dressings and reinforcement will be left intact for 24–48 hours postoperatively

Structure	Process	Outcome
S3 Ward protocols clearly state the need for the primary dressing and reinforcement to be left intact for 24–48 hours postoperatively	P3 Staff are made aware of the protocol requirements	O3 All primary donor site dressings and reinforcement are left intact for 24–48 hours postoperatively

Audit indicators	Criteria	Audit activity	Findings and comments	Compliance	
				Achieved	Expected
1	**S1** Theatre guidelines indicate moist wound-healing products should be used	Review procedural guidelines for types of dressings for donor sites	The recommended primary dressings listed were all moist wound-healing products	100%	100%
1	**P1** Moist wound-healing products should be used	Review of theatre stores for moist wound-healing products for donor sites	Moist wound-healing products were found to be readily available	100%	100%
1	**01** Moist wound-healing products are used on all donor sites	Review postoperative patient records for descriptions of types of primary dressings applied	The primary dressings applied were all moist wound-healing products	100%	100%
2	**S2** Theatre guidelines recommend dressing selection based on anticipated moisture-absorbing requirements of the primary dressing	Theatre guidelines reviewed for recommendations to include estimates of wound fluid loss in primary dressing selection	Documented estimates of size and moisture-bearing capacities required of primary dressing were not included in the guidelines	0%	100%
2	**P2** Estimated wound fluid loss is evaluated as part of the dressing selection criteria	Theatre documentation was reviewed for evidence of fluid loss estimates	No documented evidence of fluid loss estimates	0%	100%
2	**02** Type and size of primary dressing is appropriate for the estimated moisture management requirements	Frequency of strikethrough was assessed by asking nurses on the day of the audit	5 = number with strikethrough; 15 = number without strikethrough	75%	100%
3	**S3** Ward protocols clearly state the need for the primary dressing and reinforcement to be left intact for 24–48 hours postoperatively	Review of ward-based documentation and practice guidelines	No protocols or documented guidelines were identified	0%	100%
3	**P3** Ward staff are made aware of the protocol requirements	All ward nursing staff rostered on the day of the audit were asked if they knew of the protocol requirements	N/A as there were no protocols	100%	100%
3	**03** All primary donor site dressings are reinforced for a minimum of 24–48 hours postoperatively	All donor sites between 24 and 48 hours postoperatively old were visually inspected for the presence of reinforcing	Not all donor sites were left/reinforced for the first 24 hours; some were removed by patients or ward nursing staff	75%	100%

(continued)

Facility/ward: _____ Clinical auditing program: _____

Audit topic: *Split thickness skin graft donor sites: post-harvest management*   **Date:** _____
Related standards: JBI *Best Practice* information sheet 2(1) 1998
Summary of audit findings/comments and action plan

Indicator 1

Compliance/Identified problems	Action
100% compliance	No action required

Indicator 2

Compliance/Identified problems	Action
S2: 0% compliance *n* = compliant *n* = noncompliant	Staff meeting with stakeholders from theatre and ward settings to discuss and clarify the rationale for dressing selection based on estimated moisture management requirements of the primary dressing
P2: 0% compliance *n* = compliant *n* = noncompliant	Reinforcement of the role of documentation as the primary legal avenue for communication of patient care and interventions
O2: 75% compliance 15 = no strikethrough 5 = strikethrough	Strikethrough and use of additional reinforcing not found to be as significant a problem as anecdotally suggested. Ward staff to commence six weeks of data collection on rates of strikethrough, and application of additional reinforcing to clarify the scope of this problem

Indicator 3

Compliance/Identified problems	Action
S3: 0% compliance	Focus group of nursing and medical staff to develop a ward protocol for postoperative management of donor sites, which included leaving the primary dressing and reinforcing intact for 24–48 hours postoperatively
P3: 0% compliance as protocol not yet developed	
O3: 0% compliance as protocol not yet developed	

Conclusions and outcomes of audit activity

The audit indicated that moist wound-healing products were consistently used on all donor sites, achieving 100% compliance with known best practice. The audit also identified that staff were reliant on the availability of up-to-date guidelines to inform practice, and that, when such guidelines were missing or incomplete, practice became variable. This was evident in the lack of structured documentation on assessment of dressing selection and on the requirement to leave primary dressings intact for 24–48 hours postoperatively. The audit results also showed that clinical documentation does not consistently describe the required details of split thickness skin graft donor sites.

The outcomes of the practice manual review and update will be reaudited in six months' time to measure improvement in outcomes. The current results will be made available to relevant practice areas, with particular focus on the achievement of 100% compliance for audit indicator 1.

10.10 Conclusion

Nurses make patient care decisions that result in changes to practice as an expected outcome of patient assessment and care planning. When decisions to change practice are made, it is important to establish that the changes have been implemented correctly, and that the expected outcomes are being achieved. Indeed, determining whether implemented changes in care provision have actually influenced patient outcomes is a crucial step in the evidence-based cycle (Flemming & Fenton 2002) and can be undertaken through clinical audit. Moreover, as we have discussed, evaluation through clinical audit can take place before initiation of best practice or afterwards.

While clinical audit is most often cited as a tool for use in the evaluation phase of the evidence-based cycle, it is in fact an excellent tool for encouraging the implementation of best practice and generating an evidence-based culture (Shakib 2002). Through the continual review of the delivery of care and taking action to improve it when deficiencies are identified (Kinn 1995:35) clinical audit is used to develop and refine healthcare practices (Morrell & Harvey 1999). This chapter has reviewed the concept of clinical audit and its place in EBP.

An example drawn from practice has been provided as a template to audit, and other useful resources have been identified. The reader is invited, for example, to examine the Auditmaker software available from the ACEBCP website. Clinical audits require a structured approach to their design and implementation. Attention should be given to institutional approval, and, where appropriate, a multidisciplinary approach, and in all cases careful planning and rigorous implementation. All of the material provided in this chapter is designed to assist clinicians to more confidently undertake audit. In this way audit can become a part of routine healthcare, thus facilitating a process of continuous quality improvement and increased standards of care.

10.11 Discussion questions

1. Consider your own area of practice. What topic/s do you think would be suitable for a clinical audit?
2. Why are they suitable?
3. How do you think a clinical audit could improve outcomes in this area?
4. What additional skills are needed to undertake a clinical audit?
5. What barriers might impact on your ability to conduct a clinical audit?
6. How might these be overcome?

10.12 References

Australian Centre for Evidence Based Clinical Practice (ACEBCP) 2003. Viewed 11 August 2003. Available at www.acebcp.org.au/current.htm#stat.

Balogh R 1996 Exploring the links between audit and the research process. *Nurse Researcher* 3(3):5–16.

Borbasi S, Jackson D, Langford RW 2004 *Navigating the maze of nursing research: an interactive learning adventure*. Mosby, Sydney.

Burnett A, Winyard G 1998 Clinical audit at the heart of clinical effectiveness. *Journal of Quality in Clinical Practice* 18(1):3–19.

Closs S, Cheater P 1996 Audit or research: what is the difference? *Journal of Clinical Nursing* 5(4):249–56.

Department of Health (UK) 1993 *Clinical audit: meeting and improving standards in health care.* Department of Health, London.

Department of Health (UK) 2001 *The essence of care: patient-focused benchmarking for health care practitioners.* Department of Health, London.

Dickinson E 1998 Clinical effectiveness for health care quality improvement. *Journal of Quality in Clinical Practice* 18(1):37–46.

Flemming K, Fenton M 2002 Making sense of research evidence to inform decision making, in C Thompson & D Dowding (eds) *Clinical decision-making and judgement in nursing,* pp 109–29. Churchill Livingstone, Edinburgh.

Garland G, Corfield F 1999 Audit, in S Hamer & G Collinson (eds) *Achieving evidence based practice,* pp 129–49. Balliere Tindall, London.

Gaston C 2003 Governance in the South Australian public health system: briefing paper no 4, general health review, Department of Human Services. Available at www.dhs.sa.gov.au/generational-health-review/documents/Briefing%20Papers/Briefing%20No%204.pdf.

Joanna Briggs Institute (JBI) 2001 *Acute care clinical auditing manual.* JBI, Adelaide.

Johnston G, Crombie I, Davies H et al 2000 Reviewing audit: barriers and facilitating factors for effective clinical audit. *Quality in Health Care* 9(1):23–6.

Kinn S 1995 Clinical audit: a tool for practice. *Nursing Standard* 9(15):35–6.

Mason A 2002 The emerging role of clinical audits. *Clinical Medicine* 2(4):294–6.

Mead D, Moseley L 1996 Research-based measurement tools in the audit process: issues of use, validity and reliability. *Nurse Researcher* 3(3):17–34.

Morgan L, Fenessey G 1996 How to undertake clinical audit: a new service. *Nursing Standard* 10(51):32–3.

Morrell C, Harvey G 1996 Clinical audit. *Nursing Standard* 10(17):38–44.

Morrell C, Harvey G 1999 *The clinical audit handbook.* Balliere Tindall, London.

Morrell C, Harvey G, Kitson A L 1995 *The reality of practitioner based quality improvement,* report no 14. National Institute for Nursing, Oxford.

National Centre for Clinical Audit 1997 *Key points from audit literature related to criteria for clinical audit.* NCCA, London.

National Health Service Executive Clinical Effectiveness 1998 Clinical effectiveness. *Nursing Times* July:1–31.

National Institute for Clinical Excellence (NICE) 2002 *Principles for best practice in clinical audit.* Available at www.nice.org.uk/text-only.asp?page=home.htm.

Perry L 2002 Implementing best evidence in clinical practice, in J V Craig & R L Smyth (eds) *The evidence-based practice manual for nurses,* pp 240–73. Churchill Livingstone, Edinburgh.

Scally G, Donaldson L J 1998 Clinical governance and the drive for quality improvement in the new NHS in England. *British Medical Journal* 317(4 July):61–5.

Scott P V 2000 Differentiating between audit and research: clinical audit is research. *I* 320(7236, 11 March):713.

Shakib S 2003 *Auditmaker for health professional: a generic tool for clinical audit manual.* Available from the Australian Centre for Evidence Based Clinical Practice at www.acebcp.org.au/auditmaker.pdf or http://logicsquad.net/auditmaker.pdf.

Shakib S, Phillips P A 2003 The Australian Centre For Evidence-based Clinical Practice Generic Audit Tool: Auditmaker for health professionals. *Journal of Evaluation in Clinical Practice* 9(2):259–63.

Thomas B 1999 Research and audit in effective health services. *Nursing Standard* 13(33):40–2.

Thompson C, Learmonth M 2002 How can we develop an evidence-based culture?, in J V Craig & R L Smyth (eds) *The evidence-based practice manual for nurses*, pp 211–39. Churchill Livingstone, Edinburgh.

Walshe K, Spurgeon P 1997 Developing a framework for assessing and improving the effectiveness of clinical audit in the NHS. Research report to the NHS executive, August.

World Health Organization (WHO) 1983 *The principles of quality assurance.* Copenhagen, WHO (report on a WHO meeting) in Scally and Donaldson (1998).

chapter 11

Undertaking a program evaluation

Elizabeth Manias

11.1 Learning objectives

After reading this chapter, you should be able to:

1. *define important components of a program, including the goal, outcome, strategy, performance indicator and performance measure*
2. *describe the purpose of the five types of program evaluation: proactive; clarificative; interactive; monitoring; and impact, and*
3. *determine the type of program to be undertaken in terms of the questions being asked about the program and the timing of its delivery.*

11.2 Introduction

The current emphasis on evidence-based practice (EBP) and provision of quality care means that nurses need to demonstrate how their nursing-care activities work and to give rationales of why they work. Completing a program evaluation provides a formalised way of addressing this need. This chapter presents the fundamental processes involved with carrying out a program evaluation. First, it considers definitions of essential terms that are often used in program evaluations. Second, it examines five forms of evaluation that underpin evaluative activities: proactive; clarificative; interactive; monitoring; and impact. Third, the chapter provides case studies from the health literature that illustrate how these forms of evaluation are used.

11.3 Definitions

Program evaluation involves the process of conducting a systematic appraisal of a particular activity for the purpose of generating knowledge and planning future strategies. Another term that is sometimes used for program evaluation is outcomes research. A number of definitions of program evaluation exist. Green (1986:171) who refers to the importance of benchmarking defines program evaluation as comparing an activity of interest with a standard of acceptability. This definition is useful because it includes the process, impact and outcomes that can be examined, and facilitates a range of standards of acceptability. Evaluation must be congruent with the goals and objectives of the program activity and the measurement of these activities needs to be appropriate. Evaluation is also a continuous process of asking questions, thinking about the responses, and reviewing the planned strategy and activity (O'Connor & Parker 1995).

Several other parameters are important in undertaking a program evaluation, which include the program's goals, outcomes, strategies, objectives, performance indicators and performance measures. These parameters are explained in Table 11.1. These terms are interpreted in different ways. Government organisations and funding bodies often use their own specific definitions of these terms and it is important to use the definitions provided by these instrumentalities to make sure that particular components are addressed (Department of Health and Aged Care 2001).

Table 11.1 Parameters in a program evaluation

Term	Meaning
Goal	The aim that the initiative seeks to achieve in general
Outcome	The changes in attitude, behaviour, health condition or status that the initiative seeks to achieve. It also concerns the learning outcomes in relation to process, knowledge and skills
Strategy	The plan used to achieve the desired outcomes
Objective	The specific targets that need to be accomplished in an effort to achieve the outcomes
Performance indicator	The responses or measured changes in attitude, behaviour, health condition or status that indicate progress towards objectives and outcomes
Performance measure	The way in which changes in attitude, behaviour, health condition or status will be measured

11.4 Forms of program evaluation

Program evaluation is classified according to the purpose of the intended activities. There are five forms of evaluation that underpin the various roles of evaluative activities: proactive; clarificative; interactive; monitoring; and impact (Owen & Rogers 1999). Table 11.2 shows the basic elements of each form, including the purpose, focus and timing for program delivery.

Table 11.2 Evaluation forms: purpose, focus and timing

	Proactive	Clarificative	Interactive	Monitoring	Impact
Purpose of evaluation	Synthesis of program	Provide explanation	Improvement	Justification, refinement	Justification, accountability
Focus	Context of program	Development of program	Development of program	Delivery and outcome of program	Delivery and outcome of program
Timing on program delivery	Before	During	During	During	After

Source: Adapted from Owen & Rogers 1999.

11.4.1 Proactive evaluation

This form of evaluation takes place before the program commences. Its purpose is to provide evidence of what is known about the issue, and to use this information in deciding how to develop a program. It also provides managers with details on how an organisation needs to change to improve its effectiveness (Owen & Rogers 1999, Scheirer 1998).

Some of the characteristic questions of this form include:
- Is there a need for the program at all?
- What are the best practice guidelines in this area?
- What research is currently available about this problem?

Three main approaches are used with this form of analysis: needs assessment; review of available literature; and review of best practice guidelines. A needs assessment addresses the problems or conditions of a particular community or organisation that should be included in future planning. It usually occurs when individuals are concerned about the present situation and type of service delivery. This approach provides valuable information about the initiatives that could be implemented to improve the situation in the future. A needs assessment is helpful in setting priorities for healthcare and allocating scarce resources. In addressing a need of a particular program, evaluators are concerned about differences between the current and desired situations, thereby establishing discrepancies. Reasons are sought for these discrepancies and decisions can be made about which needs should be given priority for action (Roth 1990).

A review of available literature involves collating what is known about the area of inquiry. It includes an examination of research publications and systematic reviews that may have already been completed on the area of interest. Most importantly, it considers how previous research has been applied to the practice setting. After the current state of research work is described and critiqued, the review should give some indication of the gaps in knowledge on the topic.

A review of best practice guidelines requires selecting and examining exemplary practice in the area. Such an approach enables the creation of benchmarks. Benchmarking has become very prominent over recent times, as organisations such as hospitals, universities and government bodies model their activities against known leaders in their field. In establishing benchmarks, it is important to identify the area of best practice, and consider whether this practice applies to the organisation. Evaluators determine how the practice is performed, and how well it is carried out relative to the best markers. After comparisons are made, it is important for managers to determine how they want the organisation to perform, relative to exemplary practice.

Data collection methods employed in proactive evaluation involve review of documents and databases, the Delphi technique, strategic planning meetings and focus groups. Examples of documents and databases that may be reviewed include hospital data such as morbidity, mortality and length of hospital stay (Centers for Disease Control and Prevention 1999). The Delphi technique requires individuals to work independently and to pool their written ideas about a particular issue. Each individual is given a list of the collected ideas, which are formatted into a set of scaled items, and asked to assess their relative importance and relevance. Strategic planning meetings are events designed to provide direction for a projected program. Individuals involved in delivering the program collaborate to consider barriers and facilitators to achieving certain activities, what they have achieved and what they wish to achieve in the future. The focus group is a method that aims to collect information from a selected group of people. While the goal of the Delphi technique is to achieve consensus, the desired outcome of focus groups is to obtain a range of views.

Case study: review of available literature and best practice guidelines

Bucknall et al (2001) examined best practice guidelines for acute pain against past research on pain. The paper evaluated the implications of the National Health and Medical Research Council (NHMRC) acute pain guidelines on nursing practice, and addressed the inadequacies of current implementation policies of hospitals. The authors argued that the NHMRC pain management guidelines failed to decrease patients' pain because healthcare professionals, organisations and researchers largely ignored the impact of contextual issues on clinical decision making. Contextual issues included patient involvement and control, nurses' pain assessment and management skills, multidisciplinary collaboration, organisational management, educational needs and evaluation of pain effectiveness. The authors recommended that future pain management programs should consider acknowledging contextual issues in their development and implementation.

Case study: review of best practice guidelines and hospital policy

Manias (1998) examined the effectiveness of best practice guidelines for the 'Do Not Resuscitate' (DNR) hospital policy on nurses' decision making. A questionnaire was developed by the author, and distributed to nurses employed in four practice areas of six metropolitan hospitals. The practice areas included: acute medical; acute surgical; coronary care; and intensive care wards. The investigator showed that decision making was not affected by nurses' awareness or lack of awareness of a DNR policy in hospitals where a policy was present. In the study, while nurses perceived that the patient, next-of-kin and nurse should play a predominant role in the DNR decision, medical doctors were usually responsible for the DNR decision. In developing DNR programs hospital managers should implement strategies aimed at ensuring nurses, patients and next-of-kin contribute actively in the decision.

11.4.2 Clarificative evaluation

The purpose of this form of evaluation is to examine the underlying structure, rationale and function of a program. It focuses on the internal components of a program rather than the way in which the program is implemented. The need for clarification may occur when there are conflicts over components of a program's design. Individuals may also require further details about how the program activities link with intended outcomes (Owen & Rogers 1999).

Characteristic questions associated with this form of evaluation include:
- What is the rationale for this program?
- What are the intended outcomes for this program?
- What structures need to be changed to ensure that intended outcomes are achieved?

Two main approaches are used in this form of evaluation: program logic development and accreditation (Owen & Rogers 1999). Program logic development involves examining available documentation and conducting interviews with relevant stakeholders to construct an overview of what the program is intended to do. It also considers how the current program could be changed to address the intended outcomes.

Accreditation determines the worth of a particular program. In health and education arenas, it involves the process of certifying that an organisation can deliver the program activity over a particular time period. This approach provides consumers with the confidence of knowing that accredited programs are of an acceptable quality.

Data collected for clarificative evaluation usually include document analysis, interviews and observations. Document sources could involve policy statements, memoranda, hospital reports, legislation, and meeting agenda and minutes. In conducting interviews and observations, the goal is to identify the most critical elements of a program between members of the evaluation team and key program staff. The views of stakeholders are also sought and compared to the elements identified in interactions between program and evaluation staff. Decisions can then be made about how the program can be implemented.

Case study: program logic development 1

Manias et al (2000) described the benefits of combining objective and naturalistic methods when undertaking a formative evaluation of a computer-assisted learning program in pharmacology for nursing students. During the design and development phases, the pharmacology program was evaluated using observation of student pairs, student questionnaires and student focus group interviews. The combination of evaluation methods enabled complex issues underlying program effectiveness to be addressed.

> # Case study: program logic development 2
>
> Ellis and Hogard (2003) evaluated a pilot scheme for clinical facilitators in acute medical and surgical wards. The clinical facilitators were employed to address two issues: the nursing skills demonstrated by newly graduated nurses; and concerns about supervision in clinical placement. The purpose of the clinical facilitators was to enhance undergraduate nurses' competence on clinical placement. Evaluation involved a three-phase approach covering outcomes, process and multiple stakeholder views. The work of clinical facilitators was evaluated using interviews, focus groups, and questionnaires with students, clinical staff and university staff. While clinical facilitators were evaluated in a positive way, concerns were raised about communication. University staff also tended to rate the clinical facilitators less favourably than did students and clinical staff.

11.4.3 Interactive evaluation

Interactive evaluation examines the delivery and implementation of a program. As this form is particularly important for program activities that are constantly changing, it has a strong element of improving processes. Individuals are also given an opportunity to better understand how and why a program functions in certain ways. This form of evaluation does not focus on the outcomes or the end-products of the program. Key stakeholders are more interested in undertaking an evaluation that supports change and improvement (Owen & Rogers 1999).

Characteristic questions associated with this form include:
- How is the delivery of the program working?
- What is the program attempting to achieve?
- How can the delivery be changed to make program delivery more effective?
- How can the organisation be changed to make program delivery more effective?

Approaches used in interactive evaluation involve responsive evaluation, action research and quality review. Responsive evaluation involves a detailed documentation of the implementation of a program. It takes into account the views and values of various stakeholders including the providers and consumers (Guba & Lincoln 1981, 1989; Patton 1980). An evaluation is considered responsive if it is orientated more towards the activities of the program rather than its purpose or outcomes.

Action research involves an intensive and reflective process of determining whether the various methods of program delivery are making a difference. It requires the evaluator going into the environment and working with individuals as coresearchers or coevaluators, in an attempt to find solutions to problems. Solutions to problems are collaboratively decided upon, carried out and examined through reflection (Wadsworth 1990). Action research involves a cyclical, systematic process of planning, acting, observing

173

and reflecting, which subsequently leads to a revised plan, and further acting, observing and reflecting (Kemmis & McTaggart 1988).

Quality reviews take place within the organisation delivering the program. Individuals within the organisation evaluate their processes and make changes depending on initiatives developed at the wider organisational level. Individuals delivering the program usually carry out quality reviews: expertise through experienced evaluators is not usually available (Colton 1997, Owen & Rogers 1999).

Data-collection methods for responsive evaluation and quality reviews involve reflective journalling, collaborative meetings and strategic planning workshops. Methods commonly used in action research include participant observation, interviews and reflective journalling (Shortell 1999). Participants may include consumers or providers of program initiatives.

Case study: quality review

Manias and Aitken (2003) described the development, implementation and evaluation of a new critical-care nursing curriculum. It examined lecturers' and clinical educators' views, and explored students' perspectives of the old curriculum compared with the new curriculum. Three data-collection methods were used for this quality review. Comprehensive and reflective notes were kept of meetings conducted during the development and implementation of the curriculum. Focus group interviews were conducted with students before and during the introduction of the new curriculum. Anonymous quality of teaching surveys, distributed by a centralised university process, were also completed by two groups of critical-care nursing students: one before and the other following the introduction of the new curriculum. Evaluation of the development and implementation enabled the investigators to further refine the curriculum to address the challenging and competing needs of clinical educators, clinical nurses, lecturers, students and university management.

Case study: action research

Blackford et al (1997) completed a two-year participatory action research study that explored the activities of nurses caring for non-English-speaking families. A number of clinical settings of a children's hospital were involved in the study: the emergency department; the intensive care unit; the cardiac unit; the general medical unit; and the neonatal unit. Thirty-three nurses were recruited to participate as coresearchers in the study. A variety of quantitative and qualitative data collection methods were used, including small surveys, questionnaires, individual interviews and focus group interviews. Workshops were conducted to bring the nurses together in order to communicate progress and to encourage discussion. The researchers also used hospital and government policy documents in addressing their findings. For example, Guidelines for Health Agencies of the Health Department of Victoria and the Patient Dependency Audit of the hospital were consulted to determine the communicative needs of non-English-speaking clients.

Data were analysed to identify key findings, strategies and implications for practice, which informed the next round of action plans. The findings showed that nurses silenced non-English-speaking families by not providing them with supports to express themselves, or by positioning them on the margins. The culture of clients and their families was either ignored or judged against the dominant Anglo-Australian culture. Coresearching nurses developed and implemented strategic action plans, which led to improved communication. For instance, coresearchers created information packages to assist in identifying interpreter and cultural needs of non-English-speaking families. The effects of the action plans were evaluated and a number of changes in nursing practice were identified. Interpreter services reported an 85% increase in the demand for their services, and nurses became better informed about the dietary and religious needs of families.

11.4.4 Monitoring evaluation

Monitoring evaluation is applied when a program is established. Individuals are usually familiar with the goals and outcomes, and have begun to implement the program. The need to undertake this form of evaluation arises from managers who wish to determine the success of the program, analyse its effectiveness and analyse efficiencies (Grembowski 2001, Hulscher et al 1999, Owen & Rogers 1999).

Characteristic questions associated with this form of evaluation include:
- How is the program reaching its target population?
- What are the costs of implementing the program and how do these compare with expectations?
- Can the program be changed to make it more effective?
- Can the program be changed to make it more efficient?
- How is implementation of the program meeting anticipated benchmarks?

Approaches used in this form of evaluation involve component analysis, devolved performance assessment and systems analysis (Owen & Rogers 1999). Component analysis requires a systematic examination of a particular aspect of the program, which is then compared to the overall goals of the organisation and the program. In deciding upon which component to investigate, managers may consider selecting a poorly running, new or expensive intervention.

Devolved performance assessment is the process whereby individuals who work in specific departments of an organisation set up evaluation procedures that report regularly to managers about their progress. This approach involves assessing the performance of all components of a program on a regular basis. Senior managers receive these assessments and make judgments about how the components contribute to the overall mission of the organisation and goals of the program.

Systems analysis involves the central managers setting up uniform evaluation procedures that are used by all departments of the organisation. This type of approach is centrally specified and disseminated for implementation to a large number of sites. An example may include the Course Experience Questionnaire that is sent out by the Department of Education, Science and Technology to every Australian graduating university student.

Data-collection methods involve examining particular indicators, which allow judgments to be made about the quality and effectiveness of a program. Indicators are used to compare a program's trends over time, and to compare the performance of a program against an acceptable set of standards. They are also valuable for comparing the implementation of the same program at different sites. Indicators must give details about the program's appropriateness, efficiency and effectiveness. In other words, indicators should provide information about how the program's objectives match with community and government expectations, the relative cost of achieving a positive impact from the program and how the program's objectives compare with its outcomes (Owen 1993). An example of an efficiency indicator is the ratio of the number of patients from a cardiac rehabilitation program related to the cost of running such a program. Using the same example, an effectiveness indicator could involve the ratio of the number of patients who do not experience a myocardial infarction from a cardiac rehabilitation program in a given time, versus the number who have enrolled in the program.

Case study: component analysis

The Office of Statewide Health Planning and Development in California collects and disseminates financial and clinical data from licensed health facilities (Joint Commission on Accreditation of Healthcare Organizations & National Pharmaceutical Council 2003). Managers and healthcare professionals at the University of California Medical Center expanded the mandated data collection to include data obtained from pain assessment interviews and chart audits. While these data were maintained for internal use, the hospital obtained this information to provide quarterly performance information that could be used to determine trends and track effectiveness. For instance, in one particular initiative, the charts of 433 patients were reviewed. It was found that a hospital-specific documentation standard was met in only 39% of charts. A structural barrier relating to the forms used was identified, which was easily corrected to improve the score. Following this change, 217 patients were interviewed and 92% reported that pain relief action was taken within 20 minutes of their communication of pain.

11.4.5 Impact evaluation

This form of evaluation involves an analysis of an established program. While a major intent of impact evaluation is to determine outcomes, it may also examine how the program is implemented. Following the conduct of impact evaluation, a decision is made about whether the program made a difference to the groups receiving it, or whether one program was better than another. Judgments can then be made about whether to continue with an activity or to change it in some way. Impact evaluation is retrospective because it is undertaken on programs that have had sufficient time to create an effect (Grembowski 2001, Owen & Rogers 1999).

Characteristic issues of this form of evaluation include:
- How cost-effective has the program been?
- To what extent have the anticipated goals been met?
- Were any unintended outcomes apparent?
- How adequately has the program served individuals' needs?

There are four main approaches to this form of evaluation: objectives-based evaluation; process–outcomes analysis; needs-based assessment; and performance audit (Owen & Rogers 1999). An objectives-based evaluation requires examining the extent to which the stated objectives of the program have been achieved. In identifying the objectives of the program, a variety of sources may be used, including policy documents, position statements for the role of different healthcare professionals and program statements. Interviews with relevant stakeholders should be undertaken, and may include nursing students, nurses, patients and representatives of health-regulating and professional bodies (Brandon 1999). If using instrument tools to determine the transfer of program objectives into outcomes, it is important to ensure that they have been validated. If suitable instruments are not available, evaluators may need to develop new measures that accurately reflect the intention of the program.

A process–outcomes analysis involves scrutinising the way in which a program is implemented. In this approach, the focus is on how a program is put into practice, and the effect that this has on the intentions of the program. Observational techniques are the best way in which to undertake this approach.

A needs-based assessment has already been described and involves the degree to which the program meets the needs of individuals using it. The assumption made in considering this approach is that the goals of the program may not necessarily reflect the consumers' needs. A needs-based approach adopts an external standard of reference to determine a program's worth.

Finally, a performance audit involves analysing if the program actually produces expected benefits, and the cost associated with these benefits. The basic premises of a performance audit are that healthcare resources are scarce, there are insufficient resources to satisfy all wants, resources have different uses, and people have different wants (Elixhauser et al 1998, Grembowski 2001, Reid 2000, Rice 1996). The challenge involves deciding how to allocate scarce resources to satisfy individual wants. There are four ways in which cost can be evaluated in economic terms (see Table 11.3). It is important to note that economic evaluation determines the cost of a program as well as its outcomes. Organisational factors can change the effectiveness of programs. For example, cost-effectiveness varies depending on the relative cost of the clinical staff involved in implementing the program (Thorogood & Coombes 2000). Nurses and other healthcare professionals are often used in evaluation endeavours because they are cheaper to employ than doctors.

177

Table 11.3 Performance audit describing four ways of economic evaluation of programs

Type of economic evaluation	Characteristics
Cost-effectiveness analysis (CEA)	This type allows judgments to be made about the relative efficiency of alternative ways of achieving a desired benefit. A program is efficient if no other program is as effective at a lower cost
Cost–benefit analysis (CBA)	The program is considered to have value when its benefit is equal to or exceeds its costs, or the ratio of benefits to costs is equal to or greater than 1.0 for a particular program. Alternatively, the benefit/cost ratio of one program is equal to or exceeds the benefit/cost ratio of another program
Cost minimisation analysis (CMA)	Two programs are considered to have identical outcomes, and the goal of analysis is to determine which program has the lower cost
Cost utility analysis (CUA)	The outcomes of two programs are weighted by their value or quality, which is determined by a common measure, such as 'quality adjusted years'. The goal of analysis is to determine which program has the most quality-adjusted life years at lower cost

Source: Adapted from Grembowski 2001.

Cost-effectiveness also varies according to the risk level of populations involved. Thus, in some cases, interventions directed at patients at high risk are more efficient than those directed at patients at a relative low risk. In the healthcare sector, economic efficiency refers to the ability to maximise health outcomes with a given amount of resources. In determining outcomes in economic terms, the objectives of the program are reduced to measures of efficiency. This approach advocates the more efficient the program, the more worthy it is. Typically, most impact evaluations consider cost implications together with other health-related outcomes, such as quality of life, re-admission to hospital and functional ability. Table 11.3 describes the different ways in which the economic attributes of a program can be evaluated.

Impact evaluation involves the use of experimental or descriptive–exploratory research designs to test the effectiveness of a program. Examples include quasi-experimental comparative, controlled studies, randomised controlled trials and qualitative studies using observations and interviews. Validated instruments are used to test the effectiveness of a program. Document analyses of policy documents and program statements are also conducted. For process–product studies, observations and interviews are undertaken with program providers and consumers to determine whether the goals of the program have been met. The results of the evaluation are presented to the policy makers who will make rational decisions about its benefits.

Case study: process–product

Manias and Bullock (2002) examined the effectiveness of pharmacology education in undergraduate and graduate nursing programs in preparing graduate nurses for clinical practice. The study was undertaken by two university academics who had no formal collaborative links with the participating clinical nurses or hospitals. Six focus group interviews were conducted with clinical nurses at two metropolitan and two regional hospitals, in which information was sought about their perceptions and experiences of graduate nurses' pharmacology knowledge. Four themes were identified. Participants indicated that graduate nurses had enormous deficits in their pharmacology knowledge. There was an unstructured approach with addressing the continuing education needs of graduate nurses. Participants valued the importance of theoretical and clinical principles of pharmacology knowledge for safe nursing practice. Finally, they believed university undergraduate nursing education should instil a greater sense of responsibility and accountability among students in their monitoring and administering of medications. The investigators concluded that current teaching and learning opportunities at the undergraduate and graduate levels were inadequate in developing and enhancing nurses' pharmacology knowledge.

Case study: objectives-based evaluation and performance audit

Hurworth et al (1988) evaluated whether a one-day on-site program conducted for 15–16-year-old students impacted on their knowledge and skills related to pre-pregnancy. Nurses and gynaecologists at the Richmond Community Health Centre in Melbourne delivered information on issues such as contraception, drugs and fetal growth. Evaluators attended two program sessions and interviewed providers in order to clarify the intentions of the program. Providers administered a survey instrument to students before and after each program session to measure achievements and to determine students' perceptions about the information presented. Evaluators also analysed the demand for the one-day program from schools situated either within or outside the Centre's immediate area. Follow-up interviews were also conducted with teachers in the participating schools to determine their views about the program. The results showed that students obtained increased scores from all schools and that male and female students had made almost equal gains in knowledge. Teachers stated that the program helped to reinforce information presented in school.

Case study: performance audit

Stewart et al (1998) described the effectiveness of a home-based intervention on readmission, death and cost among patients with congestive cardiac failure discharged home from acute hospital care. A randomised controlled trial was implemented to determine the effectiveness of the intervention. The home-based intervention comprised a single visit by a nurse or pharmacist to facilitate effective medication management, identify early clinical deterioration and optimise medical follow-up. The effects of the home-based intervention were compared to those receiving usual postdischarge care, which comprised a review by the patient's primary care physician or cardiologist in the hospital's outpatient department within two weeks of discharge.

Forty-nine patients were randomised into the intervention group and 48 were assigned to the usual care group. During follow-up, patients in the intervention group had fewer unplanned readmissions (36 versus 63, $p = 0.03$) and fewer out-of-hospital deaths (1 versus 5, $p = 0.11$). Patients in the intervention group had fewer days of hospitalisation (261 versus 452, $p = 0.05$). The mean cost of hospital-based care was lower for the intervention group ($A3200, 95% confidence interval of $A1800 to $4600) compared with the control group ($A5400, 95% confidence interval of $A3200 to $6800); however, this difference did not reach statistical significance. The cost of implementing the intervention was $A190 per patient. The investigators concluded that while the study results were promising, further work should focus on assessing the potential improvement in patient quality of life and functional status, and should be sufficiently powered to detect significant differences in readmission and out-of-hospital death.

11.5 Conclusion

This chapter described the characteristics of five forms of evaluation: proactive; clarificative; interactive; monitoring; and impact. These provide a conceptual map for evaluators, providers, consumers and other relevant individuals about how to proceed with an evaluation activity. While it is possible to evaluate all stages of a program cycle, from design and development to implementation, it is more common to select one specific form. The type of decision made depends on the kinds of questions that need to be asked about the program and the concerns of the consumers and other stakeholders.

11.6 Discussion questions

1. Define the following terms: goal; outcome; strategy; objective; performance indicator; and performance measure.
2. Differentiate between the following forms of evaluation in terms of purpose, timing and approaches used: proactive; clarificative; interactive; monitoring; and impact evaluation.
3. Hospital Y has been running a nurse-led cardiac clinic for three years. The hospital managers wish to determine how adequately the clinic has served patients' needs and the extent to which anticipated goals have been met. Describe how an evaluation could be undertaken to address the managers' concerns.
4. University lecturers have identified that their Bachelor of Nursing curriculum is too content-laden and teacher-centred. They decide to change it to a problem-based learning approach, with the focus on student-centred needs. The lecturers wish to determine how to use the characteristics of problem-based learning in developing their new curriculum. Describe how an evaluation could be undertaken in this situation.

11.7 References

Blackford J, Street A, Parsons C 1997 Breaking down language barriers in clinical practice. *Contemporary Nurse* 69(1):15–21.

Brandon P R 1999 Involving program stakeholders in reviews of evaluators' recommendations for program revisions. *Evaluation and Program Planning* 22:363–72.

Bucknall T, Manias E, Botti M 2001 Acute pain management: the implications of scientific evidence for nursing practice in the postoperative context. *International Journal of Nursing Practice* 7:266–73.

Centers for Disease Control and Prevention 1999 Framework for program evaluation in public health. *Morbidity and Mortality Weekly Report* 48(RR–11, September):17.

Colton D 1997 The design of evaluations for continuous quality improvement. *Evaluation and the Health Professions* 20:265–85.

Department of Health and Aged Care 2001 *Evaluation: a guide for good practice.* Commonwealth of Australia, Canberra.

Elixhauser A, Halpern M, Schmier J, Luce B R 1998 Health care CBA and CEA from 1991 to 1996: an updated bibliography. *Medical Care* 36(Suppl 5):MS1–MS9.

Ellis R, Hogard E 2003 Two deficits and a solution? Explicating and evaluating clinical facilitation using consultative methods and multiple stakeholder perspectives. *Learning in Health and Social Care* 2(1):18–27.

Green L W 1986 *Community health.* Mayfied Press, St Louis.

Grembowski D 2001 *The practice of health program evaluation.* Sage Publications, Thousand Oaks.

Guba E, Lincoln Y 1981 *Effective evaluation.* Jossey-Bass, San Francisco.

Guba E, Lincoln Y 1989 *Fourth generation evaluation.* Sage Publications, London.

Hulscher M, Wensing M, Grol R et al 1999 Interventions to improve the delivery of preventative services in primary care. *American Journal of Public Health* 89:737–46.

Hurworth R E, Owen J M, Griffin L D 1988 *The impact of the Richmond Community Health Centre Pre-Pregnancy Program.* Centre for Program Evaluation, University of Melbourne, Melbourne.

Joint Commission on Accreditation of Healthcare Organizations, National Pharmaceutical Council 2003 *Improving the quality of pain management through measurement and action.* Joint Commission on Accreditation of Healthcare Organizations, Oakbrook Terrace, Illinois.

Kemmis S, McTaggart R (eds) 1988 *The action research planner.* Deakin University Press, Geelong.

Manias E 1998 Australian nurses' experiences and attitudes in the 'Do Not Resuscitate' (DNR) decision. *Research in Nursing & Health* 21:429–41.

Manias E, Aitken R 2003 Achieving collaborative workplace learning in a university critical care course. *Intensive and Critical Care Nursing* 19:50–61.

Manias E, Bullock S 2002 The educational preparation of undergraduate nursing students in pharmacology: clinical nurses' perceptions and experiences of graduate nurses' medication knowledge. *International Journal of Nursing Studies* 39:773–84.

Manias E, Bullock S, Bennett R 2000 Formative evaluation of a computer assisted learning program in pharmacology for nursing students. *Computers in Nursing* 18:265–71.

O'Connor M L, Parker E 1995 *Health promotion: principles and practice in the Australian context.* Allen & Unwin, Sydney.

Owen J M 1993 *Program evaluation: forms and approaches.* Allen & Unwin, Sydney.

Owen J M, Rogers P J 1999 *Program evaluation: forms and approaches,* international edn. Sage Publications, London.

Patton M 1980 *Qualitative evaluation methods.* Sage Publications, Beverly Hills, California.

Reid R J 2000 A cost–benefit analysis of syringe exchange programs. *Journal of Health & Social Policy* 11(4):41–57.

Rice T H 1996 Measuring health care costs and trends, in R M Anderson, T H Rice & G F Kominski (eds) *Changing the US health care system: key issues in health services, policy and management,* pp 62–80. Jossey-Bass, San Francisco.

Roth J 1990 Needs and the needs assessment process. *Evaluation Practice* 11(2):39–44.

Scheirer M A 1998 Commentary: evaluation planning is the heart of the matter. *American Journal of Evaluation* 19:385–91.

Shortell S M 1999 The emergence of qualitative methods in health services research. *Health Services Research* 34(Suppl Part 2):1083–90.

Stewart S, Pearson S, Horowitz J D 1998 Effects of a home-based intervention among patients with congestive heart failure discharged from acute hospital. *Archives of Internal Medicine* 158:1067–72.

Thorogood M, Coombes Y 2000 *Evaluating health promotion: practice and methods.* Oxford University Press, Oxford.

Wadsworth Y 1990 *Everyday evaluation on the run.* Action Research Issues Association, Melbourne.

chapter 12

Development and use of evidence-based guidelines

Sonya Osborne and Joan Webster

12.1 Learning objectives

After reading this chapter, you should be able to:

1. *identify benefits and limitations of evidence-based guidelines in nursing*
2. *discuss the limitations of evidence-based guidelines*
3. *discuss a conceptual framework for developing effective evidence-based guidelines, and*
4. *apply key principles in the development and implementation of evidence-based guidelines.*

12.2 Introduction

The purpose of this chapter is to provide an overview of development and use of evidence-based guidelines as a tool for decision making in clinical practice. Nurses have always developed and used tools to guide clinical decision making related to interventions in practice. Since Florence Nightingale (Nightingale 1860) gave us 'notes' on nursing in the late 1800s, nurses have continued to use tools, such as standards, policies and procedures, protocols, algorithms, clinical pathways and clinical guidelines, to assist them in making appropriate decisions about patient care that would eventuate in the best desired patient outcomes.

Clinical guidelines have enjoyed growing popularity as a comprehensive tool for synthesising clinical evidence and information into user-friendly recommendations for practice. Historically, clinical guidelines were developed by individual experts or groups of experts by consensus with no transparent process for the user to determine the validity and reliability of the recommendations. The acceptance of the evidence-based practice (EBP) movement as a paradigm for clinical decision making underscores the imperative for clinical guidelines to be systematically developed and based on the best available research evidence.

Clinicians are faced with the dilemma of choosing from an abundance of guidelines of variable quality or developing new guidelines. Where do you start? How do you find an existing guideline to fit your practice? How do you know if a guideline is evidence-based, valid and reliable? Should you apply an existing guideline in your practice or develop a new guideline? How do you get clinicians to use the guidelines? How do you know if using the guideline will make any difference in care delivery or patient outcomes? Whatever the choice, the challenge lies in choosing or developing a clinical guideline that is credible as a decision-making tool for the delivery of quality, efficient and effective care. This chapter will address the posed questions through an exploration of the ins and outs of evidence-based clinical guidelines from development to application to evaluation.

12.3 What are clinical guidelines?

Before getting into this chapter on evidence-based clinical guidelines, it is necessary to start with a definition of a clinical guideline to differentiate it from the myriad other tools nurses use in practice (see Table 12.1). However, it is important to keep in mind that regardless of what the tool is called (e.g. algorithm, clinical pathway), the process of their development should be equally as rigorous. Clinical guidelines are 'systematically developed statements to assist practitioner and patient decisions about appropriate healthcare for specific circumstances' (Field & Lohr 1992). The broad purpose of clinical guidelines is to aid clinicians in providing quality care and to aid in the evaluation of that care against best practice.

Table 12.1 Examples of clinical practice tools

Algorithms are clinical guidelines prepared in a flowchart format, typically describing the process and decisions, allowing for alternative pathways, involved in addressing a specific condition

Clinical pathways are typically multidisciplinary management tools based on clinical information developed in other guidelines that document the essential steps in a clinical process from hospital admission to discharge, detailing timing of interventions to achieve identified outcomes

Clinical guidelines are systematically developed statements to assist clinician and patient decisions about appropriate healthcare for specific clinical circumstances (Field & Lohr 1992)

Policies are written plans of an organisation's official position, based on the organisation's purpose and goals, on a specific health situation, intended to guide and determine decisions for improving a specific health situation

Procedures are established series of ordered steps for performing specific tasks, typically associated with an identified policy

Protocols are rigid, prescribed statements, describing in detail, how the process of the most cost-effective care for a population of patients should be conducted, usually to expedite care for routine problems

Standards are accepted discipline-based principles for patient-care processes developed to increase the probability of resulting in appropriate care

Guidelines have been promoted as one strategy for bridging the research–practice gap by translating research findings into feasible recommendations ready for integration into practice. The proliferation of guidelines in the past decade has been an attempt to address the problem of variability of inappropriate practices by gathering together in one place the best available evidence to support effective and efficient care. There is some evidence that guideline-driven care by medical, nursing and allied health professionals can be effective, in varying degrees, in changing the process and improving the outcome of care (Grimshaw & Russell 1993, Thomas et al 2003).

However, in order for guidelines to reach their full potential, they must be developed with the end user in mind, developed using systematic and rigorous processes, developed simultaneously with dissemination and implementation strategies, and evaluated regularly to keep abreast of the ever-changing healthcare environment and new knowledge. With this in mind, clinicians must also be aware that not all guidelines have been developed within the confines of the above criteria and, therefore, guidelines must be critically appraised before they are accepted for use in practice. Effective guidelines assist in clinical decision making, improving the quality of healthcare, guiding resource allocation and reducing legal risk of liability. But what is an effective guideline?

12.4 What are the characteristics of effective clinical guidelines?

Grilli et al (2000) evaluated 431 guidelines produced by professional specialty organisations between 1988 and 1998 for quality based on three dimensions: description of stakeholder involvement in development process; strategy for identifying evidence; and grading of recommendations. Only 5% of guidelines in the study met all three criteria for quality, which led to the conclusion that 'explicit methodological criteria for the production of guidelines shared among public agencies, scientific societies, and patients' associations need to be set up' (Grilli et al 2000:103).

Although there is no internationally recognised and accepted framework for the development of clinical guidelines, guideline development organisations around the world are in agreement on certain key qualities required for guidelines to be effective. These key qualities include validity, reproducibility, representativeness, flexibility, adaptability, cost-effectiveness, applicability, reliability and usefulness (Field & Lohr 1992, NHMRC 1999, SIGN 2001). These key qualities should be considered when appraising existing national clinical guidelines before adaptation to local contexts and when developing new guidelines. Guideline development methodology, and therefore guidelines, can be enhanced worldwide by the adoption of an internationally accepted conceptual framework, based on the recognised key qualities. In this way internationally accepted standards for the collection and synthesis of evidence in developing effective guidelines can be established.

In Australia, the National Health and Medical Research Council (NHMRC 1999) has incorporated recognised key qualities into nine guiding principles for effective guideline development. These nine principles have been adapted and presented as a conceptual framework for guideline development in Table 12.2.

12.4.1 Principle 1: guideline development should be outcome-focused

Guidelines should be developed with inferences about specific clinical and economic outcomes. Validity of the guideline can then be assessed on how implementation of the recommendations compares with alternative treatment or management in achieving the projected outcomes.

185

Table 12.2 Conceptual framework for guideline development

Key qualities	Guideline development principles
Valid and reproducible	Guideline development should be outcome-focused
	Guidelines should be based on best available evidence and describe the strength of the link between recommendation and outcome
	Guideline evidence should be combined using the strongest method available to determine effect on clinical outcomes
Representative	Guideline development teams should be multidisciplinary and include consumer representatives
Flexible and adaptable	Guidelines should be flexible and adaptable to local conditions
Cost-effective	Guidelines should be developed with thought to resource limits
Reliable and applicable	Guidelines should be developed with thought to the target audience
	Guidelines should be evaluated for effect, value, validity and usage
	Guidelines should be reviewed and modified regularly to incorporate new evidence

Source: Adapted from NHMRC's nine guiding principles underlying the guideline development process (NHMRC 1999).

12.4.2 Principle 2: guidelines should be based on best available evidence and describe the strength of the link between recommendation and outcome

Searching for and analysing research evidence is the most expensive and time-consuming component of evidence-based guideline development (Browman 2001), and may sometimes be an impetus for taking shortcuts in the process. Meticulous processes must be adhered to so that credibility and validity of the guideline is assured. Authority of systematic reviews of the literature depends a great deal on the care of the search (Grilli et al 2000).

In addition to a careful search for evidence, the grading of that evidence is essential to discriminate evidence-based from consensus-based recommendations (Grilli et al 2000). The effectiveness of guidelines depends on the quality of the evidence upon which they are based. Guidelines should be accompanied by explicit details on how the research was judged for level of evidence, methodological quality, relevance to the research question and applicability to the target patient population. A guide to grading the recommendations based on the strength of the link between the evidence and the recommendation should be made evident.

12.4.3 Principle 3: guideline evidence should be combined using the strongest method available to determine effect on clinical outcomes

Good quality evidence is necessary but not enough when making recommendations (NHMRC 1999). Availability of evidence from one high-level study does not immediately mean a good clinical recommendation will result due to issues such as small effect size or the use of non-clinical outcomes (NHMRC 1999). In addition, one of the difficulties in searching the literature is determining effect size where there is conflicting evidence. Where more than one study is available, appropriate combination of results into a meta-analysis

186

may yield a truer picture of treatment effect. The guideline development team must be able to assess and combine not only the effect of interventions, but also the feasibility of implementation relevant to resources, and inequities that may arise in certain populations gaining access to the recommended treatment (NHMRC 1999).

12.4.4 Principle 4: guideline development teams should be multidisciplinary and include consumer representatives

Guideline development teams should be diverse and representative of all stakeholders (e.g. medical officers, nurses, allied health professionals, consumers, policy makers, health facility managers and pharmacists). A representative team can engage in a more holistic discussion of all aspects of a topic, such as relevant outcomes, patient values and barriers to implementation, instead of writing the guideline from one perspective. Involvement of all relevant stakeholders will improve the quality and continuity of care and improve the likelihood of uptake of guideline recommendations by all (NHMRC 1999). Care must be taken in assembling the guideline development team and systems should be in place so that all team members have adequate input into decision-making processes.

12.4.5 Principle 5: guidelines should be flexible and adaptable to local conditions

Local adaptation of existing guidelines is necessary to ensure the guidelines meet the quality, validity and applicability issues in the immediate setting. The NHMRC recommends that national guidelines must be flexible and amenable to local adaptation by:
• providing evidence of relevance to different target populations, different geographic settings and different clinic settings
• considering resource implications, including costs and benefits, and
• providing a way to incorporate patient values and preferences (NHMRC 1999).

12.4.6 Principle 6: guidelines should be developed with thought to resource limits

Clinical guidelines should be mindful of resource implications and provide an economic analysis of consequences if the guideline recommendations are used and if they are not used. When adapting guidelines for the local setting, consideration should be given to several factors, such as alternative treatment options, availability of equipment, variability in education, knowledge and skill, and availability of clinicians to follow through on recommendations (NHMRC 1999). Knowledge of the economic analyses will be useful in the clinicians' decision-making process to follow the guideline recommendations or choose an alternative course of action, depending on the above-mentioned factors.

12.4.7 Principle 7: guidelines should be developed with thought to the target audience

The target audience or end users of the guideline should be considered when developing strategies to disseminate and implement guideline recommendations. The target audience includes not only clinicians who will be involved in implementation of care recommendations, but also patients who will be recipients of that care. Guidelines are only as effective as their awareness, understanding and use in practice allow. The guideline must be introduced to the target audience through targeted dissemination and education strategies in conjunction with proactive strategies for overcoming barriers to uptake and use.

12.4.8 Principle 8: guidelines should be evaluated for effect, value, validity and usage

Clinical effectiveness of guidelines depends on resolution of identified problems that are the focus of the guideline. Therefore, health outcomes must be monitored after guideline implementation to determine the impact of the guideline. The impact of the guideline on clinician knowledge and practice behaviour must also be evaluated to obtain a clearer picture of the use of the guideline in practice. It is important that the guideline be evaluated for perceptions of relevance and importance to clinicians and patients, as this will have an impact on compliance with guideline recommendations.

12.4.9 Principle 9: guidelines should be reviewed and modified regularly to incorporate new evidence

Clinical guidelines become obsolete in the face of new evidence and must therefore be regularly reviewed and modified. Using the evidence-based approach to guideline development creates a solid foundation for subsequent review because any subsequent review should not have to be entirely redone, but updated from the point of the last review (Browman 2001). Shekelle et al (2001) estimate that the average 'life span' of a guideline is three years; however, more frequent updates using rigorous methods may be easier to accomplish and more valid than infrequent updates that compromise rigour to make up for lost time (Browman 2001).

12.5 How should clinical guidelines be used in practice?

The purpose of evidence-based guidelines is to assist practitioners in providing quality care by serving as a useful aid for clinical decision making (Field & Lohr 1992). The use of guidelines in conjunction with clinician expertise and judgment, and knowledge of the patient, enables clinicians to make clinical decisions that incorporate best practice into individual patient care. Guidelines are useful in assessing and assuring the quality of care (Field & Lohr 1992) and establishing best practice (Keogh & Courtney 2001). Evaluation of quality of care is enhanced by using the guideline as a framework for comparison of current practice with best practice. In this way, guidelines may also be useful in reducing risk of legal liability or negligence (Field & Lohr 1992) by establishing standards for best practice that a reasonable clinician would follow in light of the evidence available.

Guidelines are also useful in allocation of resources and the reduction of healthcare costs (Field & Lohr 1992, Keogh & Courtney 2001). Guidelines can identify recommendations for appropriate and cost-effective management of clinical conditions. Guidelines are also useful in streamlining processes (Keogh & Courtney 2001), which contributes to the best use of available resources. So, how do you use these evidence-based guidelines for practice?

12.5.1 Finding existing guidelines

Clinical guidelines can readily be found in print and electronic form, although a wider search can be made electronically with today's easy access to the World Wide Web. Electronically searching for clinical guidelines may involve a variety of resources. These include general guideline database archives (e.g. US National Guidelines Clearinghouse); specialty guideline database archives (e.g. Royal College of Nursing clinical guidelines site); citation databases (e.g. CINAHL, Medline and EMBASE); and internet search engines (e.g. Google). General and specialty-specific guideline archive databases are produced and maintained by hundreds of organisations around the world. A brief list of guideline development organisations can be found in Table 12.3. Internet search engines are also numerous and differ in their strategy for searching, the options available and the coverage offered (McSweeney et al 2001). A use of a combination of the above resources will result in a considerable amount of information; therefore, a targeted search strategy and quality filtering strategy will increase the chances of retrieving only relevant and useful guidelines.

Table 12.3 Guideline resources

Resource	Country of origin	Available at
National Health and Medical Research Council (NHMRC)	Australia	www.health.gov.au/nhmrc/publications/cphome.htm
National Health Service National Institute for Clinical Excellence (NICE)	United Kingdom	www.nice.org.uk/article.asp?a=6834
Agency for Healthcare Research and Quality (AHRQ)	United States	www.ahcpr.gov/clinic/cpgsix.htm
Canadian Medical Association (CMA) Infobase	Canada	http://mdm.ca/cpgsnew/cpgs/index.asp
Guidelines International Network (GIN)	International	www.g-i-n.net/
Joanna Briggs Institute	Australia	www.joannabriggs.edu.au/pubs/best_practice.php
New Zealand Guidelines Group (NZGG)	New Zealand	www.nzgg.org.nz
Registered Nurses Association of Ontario	Canada	www.rnao.org/bestpractices/index.asp
Royal College of Nursing (RCN)	UK	www.rcn.org.uk/resources/guidelines.php
Scottish Intercollegiate Guidelines Network (SIGN)	United Kingdom	www.sign.ac.uk/guidelines/index.html
US National Guidelines Clearinghouse	United States	www.guideline.gov/

To put the quantity of clinical guidelines in perspective, an electronic search of Medline, CINAHL and the Cochrane Library using the search term 'guideline' resulted in 6218 hits. Similarly, a search on the search engine Google using the term 'clinical guideline' resulted in 360,000 hits. The potential amount of information available should serve as an imperative for having a strategy for quickly evaluating the context and content of the guideline. In other words, how can you assess the quality of a guideline?

12.5.2 Appraising existing guidelines

As mentioned earlier in this chapter, availability of an existing guideline does not guarantee its quality, validity or applicability. Several specialty organisations may produce guidelines for the same clinical issue but offer different recommendations for practice. Whose recommendations should you follow, if any? Just as principles have been described for developing guidelines, similar principles must be used in evaluating the quality of existing guidelines. Fortunately, the principles of guideline development can also be applied to guideline evaluation.

Several critical appraisal evaluation checklists are available to help in considering application of a guideline in practice (Hayward et al 1995a, 1995b, the AGREE Collaboration 2001). One example of a guideline appraisal checklist is the 'Appraisal of guidelines, research and evaluation' (AGREE) instrument, a generic guideline appraisal checklist (the AGREE Collaboration 2001). The AGREE instrument is a user-friendly tool that focuses on six domains: scope and purpose; stakeholder involvement; rigour of development; clarity and presentation; applicability; and editorial independence. The AGREE domains can be superimposed upon the previously presented conceptual framework for guideline development to demonstrate that the same criteria for developing guidelines can and should be used to evaluate guidelines for use.

In light of the amount of information you may find through an electronic search, there must be a way to 'weed out' more useful and relevant guidelines for retrieval and further assessment. Three simple questions, which are the basis of most appraisal checklists (Ciliska et al 2001, Hayward et al 1995a, 1995b, McSweeney et al 2001), can be asked: What are the recommendations? Are the recommendations valid? Will the recommendations help me in caring for my patients?

> Busy clinicians might hope that criteria for appraising practice guidelines would obviate the need for reviewing how the guideline developers have brought together the evidence, and how they have chosen the values reflected in their recommendations. Unfortunately, any shortcuts that bypass at least a cursory look at evidence and values will leave the clinician open to being misled by guidelines that may be based on a biased selection of evidence, a skewed interpretation of that evidence, or an idiosyncratic set of values (Hayward et al 1995a:571).

A word of caution . . . in appraising guidelines for quality, validity and applicability, attention must be given to the fact that guideline recommendations are influenced by the values of the organisation producing the guideline in relation to the objective of having an effect on how clinicians practice. So, how do you decide whether to adapt an existing guideline or develop a new one?

12.5.3 Adapting existing guidelines for local use or developing new guidelines

Guideline development can be a costly, resource-intensive and time-consuming undertaking. It may better suit the needs of the organisation, team or individual to make use of the work of others, particularly national guideline development bodies and specialty organisations, instead of 'reinventing the wheel'. There are advantages and disadvantages to both approaches, although the most resource-sparing venture is to adapt existing guidelines. Regardless of the approach taken, whether adapted from national guidelines or developed locally, uptake of evidence-based guidelines is enhanced if the guideline is disseminated in user-friendly formats such as algorithms, clinical pathways, policies and procedures, standards or protocols for practice.

The main disadvantages of developing guidelines from scratch are the large investment in resources, time constraints that may negatively affect the process, and the need to hire or train clinicians in guideline development processes, small group leadership and facilitation, and information management. However, advantages of developing guidelines at the local level include capacity building in EBP, and improved uptake, use and evaluation of the guideline recommendations because of a cultural sense of 'ownership'.

As mentioned previously, local adaptation of existing guidelines is necessary to ensure the guidelines meet the quality, validity and applicability issues in the immediate setting. When adapting existing guidelines, the starting point should be a high-quality guideline. The existing guideline should have the same focus as the topic of local need and the guideline should be assessed using the same conceptual framework for developing a guideline. So, what is involved in the process of developing clinical guidelines?

12.6 How are guidelines developed?

The quality of the guideline development process influences the likely use of the guidelines in practice. The way in which guidelines are developed strongly influences their acceptance and the extent to which they are subsequently used (Field & Lohr 1992, Grimshaw et al 1995, Pagliari & Grimshaw 2002). There is international consensus by national guideline development agencies that the principles of EBP influence the development of guidelines (Burgers et al 2003). Steps in guideline development thus mimic steps in the EBP process (see Ch 1 for a review of the EBP process). These steps include: selection and focus of the topic; systematic search for scientific evidence; critical review and synthesis of best evidence into recommendations; application and implementation of the guideline in practice; and evaluation of the guideline for compliance, efficiency and effectiveness. Each of these steps will be explained in more detail below, and the process is summarised in Figure 12.1.

12.6.1 Select and focus the topic

Before embarking on the resource-intensive journey of developing a clinical practice guideline, the topic is selected and focused, and the project scoped. Usually, there is local *anecdotal* evidence of the need for a guideline on a particular topic to address variability in practice and improve patient outcomes.

191

Figure 12.1 Guideline development process

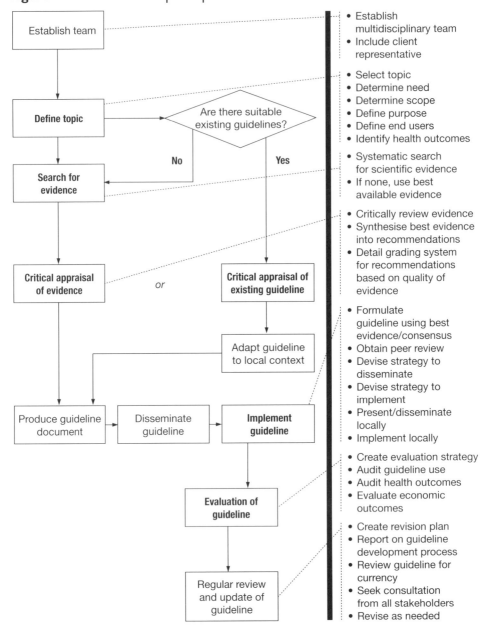

Some preliminary work must be conducted to determine whether there is *authentic* evidence to support the need. Topics are amenable to guidelines if there is uncertainty about appropriate practice, if there is variation in practice among clinicians, and if there are significant cost benefits in changing practice, without sacrificing effectiveness (Webster et al 1999).

The guideline topic can be focused using the same methods for formulating clinical questions in the EBP process (see Ch 1), whereby the patient or population with a specific health condition, as well as measurable health outcomes, are identified.

Once this preliminary work is complete a guideline development team must be established to progress the project. Ideally, this multidisciplinary team should be comprised of representatives from all stakeholder groups, such as nursing, medicine and allied health, and especially including a patient or consumer representative. Another valuable member of the team is a health science librarian and at least one member trained and experienced in critical appraisal of research.

One of the first responsibilities of the guideline development team is to come to an agreement on the purpose of the guideline, the end users or target audience, the context of guideline use, the condition or problem of focus, and the measurable outcomes that the guideline will address. A health outcome is a change in health status as a result of the appropriate choice of interventions by the healthcare provider (Donabedian 1992, NHMRC 1999). Examples of outcome measures recognised by the NHMRC include general health status, early or late morbidity, treatment complications, mortality, relapse or readmission rates, complication rates, return to work, physical and social functioning, quality of life and patient satisfaction (NHMRC 1999).

It is important for the guideline development team to be clear about the focus of the guideline, especially the problem and the outcomes, as this will not only serve as the basis for evaluation down the track, but it will immediately inform and guide the search for evidence.

12.6.2 Systematically search for scientific evidence

In order to ensure that the guideline is based on the best research evidence available, a systematic search of the literature is conducted. A properly conducted and reported systematic review creates a solid foundation for recommendations that are as current as practical (Browman 2001). Formulation of a comprehensive search strategy, using the relevant terms, is the first step in conducting a systematic search. The second step is searching the relevant literature, which includes searching electronic databases such as CINAHL, Medline and EMBASE, hand searching relevant journals, searching proceedings from relevant conferences and consulting with any other professional organisations or experts in the field who may be aware of unpublished research. The search strategy is defined not only by the patient group and outcomes under consideration, but also by the type of study design used to answer the question.

Guidelines typically are concerned with best treatment or intervention alternatives. Therefore, using a hierarchical ranking of the quality of the research for intervention studies, a systematic review of all randomised controlled trials is at the top of the evidence pyramid, followed by a well-conducted randomised controlled trial. In the absence of randomised controlled trials for intervention studies, other types of evidence from other study designs may be used to guide recommendations (see Chs 2–4 for a review of types of evidence and types of study designs).

Several guideline development organisations have suggested the use of an evidence table or balance sheet to manage the evidence collection process (NHMRC 1999, SIGN 2001). An example of an evidence table can be found on the SIGN website. In the absence of available research studies, expert opinion and consensus are other sources of evidence, albeit not as strong as evidence obtained from well-designed research studies. In any case, a transparent process for ranking the evidence based on type of study design, quality of study evidence, and strength of recommendation should be made explicit in the guideline. Credibility of the guideline recommendations depends on the quality of the evidence and the explicit link between the research evidence and the recommendations.

12.6.3 Critically review and synthesise best evidence into recommendations

Once the evidence is gathered, the next task is to critically appraise the evidence and synthesise the best evidence into recommendations. Well-constructed guideline documents contain explicit descriptions about the level of evidence used as support, how the quality of the evidence was determined and how the strength of the recommendation was established. The level of evidence is based on the study design (e.g. a randomised controlled trial). The quality of the evidence is based on the appropriateness of the study design to answer the study question and the validity of the findings. The key to critical appraisal is to use a systematic method for examining key aspects of the study in order to make an informed judgment about the quality, validity and applicability of the study (see Chs 6–8 for a review of critical appraisal techniques). It is also important to be able to synthesise the evidence in the most appropriate way (e.g. meta-analysis or metasynthesis) to determine the effect of the interventions. Several methods and tools for critically appraising specific study designs and combining study results are freely available on the World Wide Web by organisations who provide education in EBP and develop evidence-based guidelines (see Table 12.3 above).

The process of formulating recommendations from the available evidence is not always straightforward, despite systems in place for grading quality. Study quality and results can potentially be interpreted in different ways by different members of the guideline development team. In addition, there may be insufficient research available, in which case the guideline development team must be forced to rely on recommendations based on expert consensus. The team must, therefore, have simple systems in place to obtain consensus of the recommendations and it must be made explicit whether the recommendations are evidence-based or consensus-based. Once the evidence to support recommendations is obtained, it can be incorporated into the guideline document. This document should outline the entire guideline development process from the need for the guideline to the way the guideline will be evaluated for effectiveness.

12.6.4 Apply and implement the guideline

Guidelines do not implement themselves (Field & Lohr 1992). Just because a clinical guideline is available does not guarantee its uptake in practice. In order for clinical guidelines to be effective, they must be perceived as useful and they must be used.

> [Clinicians] will criticize new guidelines for novelty, old ones for age, complicated guidelines for complexity, brief guidelines for simplicity, broad guidelines for lack of specificity, narrow ones for depth, visual guidelines for over-simplicity and written guidelines for verbosity (Dowswell et al 2001:122).

194

Strategies for dissemination and implementation of clinical guidelines depend on the local setting and the target audience (NHMRC 1999). A well-designed dissemination and implementation strategy is crucial to the successful uptake and use of guidelines in practice. The guideline must be 'marketed' to the end users—clinicians as well as patients. Dissemination of new guidelines should be accompanied by targeted education programs on when and how to use the guideline. A well-conceived strategy that acknowledges possible barriers to implementation, as well as strategies to overcome or minimise those barriers is crucial to successful guideline implementation in practice. Implementation attempts incorporating patient-specific reminders aimed at specific clinicians are more likely to be associated with changed behaviour; and multifaceted implementation is associated with increased guideline use (Dowswell et al 2001). Examples of strategies that may be used for dissemination and implementation include:

- producing short summaries, printed and web-based
- incorporating the guidelines into local quality improvement processes
- presenting the guideline in user-friendly formats, such as algorithms
- piloting draft guidelines and incorporating feedback into the final document
- offering feedback on health outcomes and compliance rates
- involving end users in the development process
- using the media to publicise the completed guideline
- submitting press releases or articles to professional journals
- soliciting public endorsement of respected clinical leaders
- providing economic incentives, and
- using the educational processes of the organisation, local universities and professional organisations (NHMRC 1999).

12.6.5 Audit and evaluate the guideline in practice

Strategies for evaluation should be developed early in the guideline development process, as the success of a clinical guideline will be determined not only by the rigour of its development but by its actual use in practice.

> *The guideline development team should at least consider the connection between the goals and recommendations of the guidelines and the organisational structures and processes which might be used to measure the impact of the guidelines after implementation (Glasziou & Pirozzo 2003).*

Formulation of an evaluation and revision strategy will make the business of regular evaluation and updating of clinical guidelines less stressful. This information should be included in the report of the guideline so that the strategy can be followed consistently for subsequent revisions. Local peer review of the guideline document as well as guideline use in practice will enhance a sense of ownership and ultimate uptake of the guideline recommendations. The life span of a clinical guideline is dependent not only on prior evaluations, but also on new research and development. Therefore, regular revision is essential to ensure currency of the evidence-based recommendations.

12.7 Conclusion

This chapter has provided a process for guideline development and use. Clinical guidelines are available to assist clinicians in decision making, but should be used as an aid in conjunction with clinical expertise and judgment and knowledge of the patients' values and preferences. To be of value, guideline recommendations should give clear-cut, practical advice about a specific health condition. They must be outcome-focused and evidence-based. Guidelines must be valid, reproducible, representative, flexible, adaptable, cost-effective, applicable, reliable and useful.

Clinical guidelines will always be susceptible to criticism and will never please all clinicians all the time (Dowswell et al 2001). Even a guideline developed using a rigorous and systematic method will not be suitable for all patients with the health condition of interest because of individual patient variables. Therefore, evidence-based guidelines should not be considered the 'be all or end all', but should be viewed as a sound first step in the evidence-based management of healthcare.

12.8 Discussion questions

1. Describe six key qualities of effective guidelines.
2. What are the nine guiding principles of guideline development?
3. Discuss a strategy for finding and appraising an existing clinical guideline.
4. What are the advantages and disadvantages of developing guidelines from scratch?
5. The guideline development process has been likened to the EBP process. Discuss the steps in the process relative to guideline development.

12.9 References

AGREE Collaboration 2001 *Appraisal of guidelines for research & evaluation (AGREE) instrument,* September 2001. Retrieved 6 July 2003, from www.agreecollaboration.org/.

Browman G P 2001 Development and aftercare of clinical guidelines. The balance between rigor and pragmatism. *JAMA: Journal of the American Medical Association* 286(12):1509–11.

Burgers J S, Grol R, Klazinga N S et al 2003 Towards evidence-based clinical practice: an international survey of 18 clinical guideline programs. *International Journal for Quality in Health Care* 15(1):31–45.

Ciliska D, Cullum N, Marks S 2001 Evaluation of systematic reviews of treatment or prevention interventions. *Evidence-based Nursing* 4(4):100–4.

Donabedian A 1992 The role of outcome in quality assessment and assurance. *Quality Review Bulletin* 18(11):356–60.

Dowswell G, Harrison S, Wright J 2001 Clinical guidelines: attitudes, information processes and culture in English primary care. *International Journal of Health Planning and Management* 16:107–24.

Field M J, Lohr K N (eds) 1992 *Guidelines for clinical practice. From development to use.* National Academy Press, Washington DC.

Glasziou P, Pirozzo S 2003 (last update February 2003) *Introduction to the clinical practice development process.* Retrieved 27 August 2003, from www.health.qld.au/cdp.

Grilli R, Magrini N, Penna A et al 2000 Practice guidelines developed by specialty societies: the need for a critical appraisal. *Lancet* 355(9198):103.

Grimshaw J M, Eccles M, Russell I 1995 Developing clinically valid practice guidelines. *Journal of Evaluation in Clinical Practice* 1:37–48.

Grimshaw J M, Russell I T 1993 Effect of clinical guidelines on medical practice: a systematic review of rigorous evaluation. *Lancet* 342(8883):1317–22.

Hayward R S A, Wilson M C, Tunis S R 1995a Users' guides to the medical literature. VIII. How to use clinical practice guidelines. A. Are the recommendations valid? *JAMA: Journal of the American Medical Association* 274:570–4.

Hayward R S A, Wilson M C, Tunis S R et al 1995b Users' guides to the medical literature. VIII. How to use clinical practice guidelines. B. What are the recommendations and will they help you in caring for your patients? *JAMA: Journal of the American Medical Association* 274(20):1630–2.

Keogh S J, Courtney M 2001 Developing and implementing clinical practice tools: the legal and ethical implications. *Australian Journal of Advanced Nursing* 19(2):14–19.

McSweeney M, Spies M, Cann C J 2001 Finding and evaluating clinical practice guidelines. *The Nurse Practitioner* 26(9):30–49.

National Health and Medical Research Council (NHMRC) 1999 *A guide to the development, implementation and evaluation of clinical practice guidelines.* Commonwealth of Australia, Canberra.

Nightingale F 1860 *Notes on nursing. What it is, and what it is not.* Appleton and Company, New York.

Pagliari C, Grimshaw J M 2002 Impact of group structure and process on multidisciplinary evidenced-based guideline development: an observational study. *Journal of Evaluation in Clinical Practice* 8(2):145–53.

Scottish Intercollegiate Guidelines Network (SIGN) 2001 *A guideline developers' handbook.* Retrieved 9 September 2003, from www.sign.ac.uk/guidelines/fulltext/50/.

Shekelle P G, Ortiz E, Rhodes S et al 2001 Validity of the Agency for Healthcare Research and Quality clinical practice guidelines: how quickly do guidelines become outdated? *JAMA: Journal of the American Medical Association* 286(12):1461–7.

Thomas L, Cullum N, McColl E et al 2003 Guidelines in professions allied to medicine. *The Cochrane Library* 1:1–43.

Webster J, Lloyd W C, Pritchard M A et al 1999 Development of evidence-based guidelines in midwifery and gynaecology nursing. *Midwifery* 15:2–5.

part five ◎———•

Measurement of nursing health outcomes

chapter 13

Instruments for measuring symptoms

Patsy Yates

13.1 Learning objectives

After reading this chapter, you should be able to:

1. *discuss the significance of symptoms to nursing research and practice*
2. *identify conceptual and methodological issues to be considered in measuring symptoms*
3. *describe key dimensions of a comprehensive approach to measurement of symptoms*
4. *examine the psychometric properties of commonly used instruments for measuring symptoms, and*
5. *discuss potential areas for future research into measuring symptoms.*

13.2 Introduction

Symptoms can be defined as 'subjective experience[s] reflecting changes in the biopsychosocial functioning, sensations, or cognition of an individual' (Dodd et al 2001a). Symptoms are a core concern for nurses working in a variety of practice settings for several reasons. They can signal a change in functioning and thereby represent a major reason for seeking healthcare (Dodd et al 2001a). Moreover, nurses today care for an increasing number of older persons and individuals who are living with chronic health conditions, many of which are characterised by complex symptom profiles. For example, a recent population survey of 17,543 individuals randomly selected from the adult Australian population reported that chronic pain (defined as pain experienced every day for three months in the six months prior to interview) was reported by 17.1% of males and 20.0% of females (Blyth et al 2001). A significant body of evidence demonstrates that such symptoms have numerous distressing and debilitating effects, and that they can pose substantial social and financial burdens on the individual and the community (Blyth et al 2001).

Many aspects of symptom experiences are directly amenable to nursing intervention, and are widely acknowledged in the nursing literature as being 'nursing-sensitive outcomes'. That is, symptoms are based on the nurses' scope and domain of practice, and there is good empirical evidence linking nursing inputs and interventions to an outcome (i.e. improved symptom experiences) (Doran 2003:vii). For example, one meta-analyses of 10 years of nursing research studies from 1981–90 on teaching interventions and symptom management for patients with cancer reported strong evidence for combined intervention effectiveness (Smith & Stullenbarger 1995). Moreover, other clinical studies have reported that systematic use of structured symptom assessment can forestall increased symptom distress over time (Mercadante et al 2000).

In this chapter, we review key conceptual and methodological issues associated with measurement of symptoms in nursing research. Commonly used instruments to measure symptoms including pain and fatigue, as well as instruments for measuring symptom status in general, are also reviewed.

13.3 Issues in measuring symptoms

Like other physiological, psychological and social constructs in nursing research, measurement of symptoms requires that instruments used be valid, reliable, feasible and clinically useful. However, the measurement of symptoms poses a number of unique challenges that need to be considered when selecting an appropriate instrument for use in the research or clinical setting.

13.3.1 Multidimensionality

Symptoms are typically conceptualised as being multidimensional, comprising an individual's perception (whether a person notices a change in the way he or she usually feels), evaluation (one's judgment about the severity, cause, treatability and the effect of symptoms on their lives), as well as responses to the symptom (their physical, psychological, sociocultural and behavioural pain components) (Dodd et al 2001a). Evaluation of the symptom thus entails a complex set of factors, including intensity, location, temporal nature, frequency and affective impact. This evaluation differs to perception, which involves a higher level cognitive process of attaching meaning to the symptom (Dodd et al 2001a).

Evaluation and perception of a symptom can be influenced by a range of personal, environmental and health or illness-related variables, including demographic, psychological, sociological and physiological factors. To give just one example, research demonstrates gender differences in reports of pain (Keogh & Herdenfelt 2002) and responses to pain therapies (Pleym et al 2003). Similarly, studies indicate that experiences of dyspnoea vary according to the underlying pathology and aetiology of the symptom (Caroci Ade & Lareau 2004).

Despite the theoretical importance of the multiple dimensions to individual symptoms, much of the focus of clinical research to date has been on achieving improvements to a single dimension of a symptom. Most commonly, this dimension has been ratings of symptom severity (Gift et al 2003). This is despite the fact that in practice, nursing intervention is often targeted at addressing a broader range of dimensions, such as minimising the restrictions imposed by symptoms, or improving perceived control over one's symptoms. These broader dimensions may be influenced by, but not directly related to, changes in ratings of symptom severity. Corner and Bailey (2001) are especially critical of the dominance of the biomedical model in symptom control, arguing it is based on a limited conceptualisation of an individual's symptom experience. They suggest that a more meaning-centred approach to understanding and responding to symptoms is required.

The multidimensionality of the symptom experience suggests that a comprehensive assessment may require measurement of characteristics including: symptom occurrence, frequency and duration; symptom severity or intensity; symptom impact in terms of distress and disability; the meaning assigned to the symptom; responses to the symptom; strategies applied to manage the symptoms and the perceived effectiveness of the strategies; and factors that aggravate or alleviate the symptoms (Dodd et al 2001a). At the very least, multidimensionality requires that the nurse is cognisant of the specific aspects of the symptom experience that are being assessed by the instrument that is being used.

13.3.2 Subjectivity

Symptoms are inherently subjective. They are experienced or felt by the person themselves. While there may be a range of physiological or observational parameters that can be indicative of a symptom, such parameters are not always directly associated with a patient's perceptions and reports of their symptom experience (McCaffery & Pasero 1999). For example, degree of anaemia is not always directly related to fatigue experiences. Moreover, studies suggest that patients, nurses and caregivers vary in their ratings of symptoms (Nekolaichuk et al 1999), and that while proxies can reliably report on observable symptoms, agreement is poorest for subjective aspects of the patient's experiences such as pain, anxiety and depression (McPherson & Addington-Hall 2003).

The major implication of the subjective nature of symptoms is that the gold standard for measuring them is the person's self-report. The measurement of symptoms in people who are cognitively impaired or who are unable to describe their experiences is therefore especially problematic.

13.3.3 Dynamism

Symptom experiences will often constantly change in response to a wide range of clinical, personal and environmental factors. For example, patterns of fatigue in patients undergoing treatment for cancer are known to be associated with factors associated with the treatments themselves (Schwartz et al 2000), while the nature of the relationship between health professionals and the person with symptoms may influence how that individual reports and expresses that symptom experience. A key issue in symptom measurement is, therefore, how, when and under what circumstances should one assess an individual's symptom experience?

The implications of the dynamic nature of the symptom experience is that researchers and clinicians require an understanding of the patterns and trajectory of a specific symptom, as well as factors influencing that experience, if an accurate interpretation is to be made of the clinical relevance and significance of that symptom to the individual.

13.4 Instruments for measuring symptoms

A vast range of instruments for measuring symptoms has emerged in the literature. These instruments can be characterised as instruments that measure multiple symptoms, or instruments that measure individual symptoms. Additionally, the instruments can be characterised according to whether they assess multiple or single dimensions of symptoms. In this section, a number of commonly used instruments for measuring symptoms are reviewed.

While the focus of this chapter is instruments that have been designed solely for the purpose of measuring symptoms, it should be acknowledged that measurement of symptom experiences is also often included as a component of quality-of-life assessments. That is, in many health-related quality-of-life measures, symptoms are conceptualised as being a core domain of quality of life. Many generic and disease-specific quality-of-life instruments therefore include symptom subscales. For example, the Short Form 36 (SF–36) measure (Ware & Sherbourne 1992) comprises subscales to measure bodily pain, while the European Organization of Research and Treatment on Cancer QLQ–30 measure (Aaronson et al 1993) comprises three subscales assessing fatigue, nausea and vomiting, and pain. A comprehensive review of quality-of-life instruments is included in Chapter 14. They will therefore not be addressed in this chapter, which focuses more on a review of instruments designed primarily for the purpose of symptom assessment.

To assist in evaluating the usefulness of the instruments reviewed in this section, the following dimensions are considered:

- *Reliability.* This is the extent to which measurements are consistent and reproducible across items, individuals or occasions.
- *Validity.* This is whether an instrument measures what it is supposed to measure, accurately reflecting the domains and dimensions of the concept (e.g. whether the symptoms measured reflect the core problems experienced by the population being assessed).
- *Responsiveness.* This is the instrument's sensitivity to changes in the level of the concept being measured (e.g. whether a qualitative change in a patient's experience is detected by changes to a measurement scale) (Pringle & Doran 2003).

These dimensions assess the essential psychometric properties that need to be considered in selecting measurement instruments for research and clinical practice. In addition, the usefulness of the instrument to research and clinical practice will also be considered in this review. That is, factors such as the clinical populations and contexts for which the instrument can be used (e.g. cross-cultural applicability and relevance to different disease groups), and the practicality and feasibility of using the instrument (e.g. timing, complexity, scoring methods), will be discussed.

13.4.1 Instruments assessing multiple symptoms

Comprehensive overviews of instruments for measuring symptoms associated with various diseases and conditions can be found in several references (Bowling 1995, Frank-Stromborg & Olsen 2004, Doran 2003). The majority of these multisymptom scales have been developed for use with people with cancer, although instruments have been developed for a wide range of conditions, including respiratory disease, neurological conditions, rheumato-logical conditions, cardiovascular disease, HIV, inflammatory bowel disease and menstrual symptoms (Bowling 1995, Doran 2003). A selection of the more commonly used instruments is reviewed in the following section, and is summarised in Table 13.1.

Table 13.1 Characteristics of two instruments for assessing multiple symptoms

Instrument	Dimensions examined	Length	Administration	Scoring
Symptom Distress Scale (McCorkle & Young 1978); modified by Sutcliffe-Chidgey & Holmes (1996)	Nausea, appetite, insomnia, pain, fatigue, bowel, concentration, appearance, breathing, outlook, cough, intimate relationships with their	13 items	Self-administered Verbal instructions not essential prior to administration	Items rated on 5-point numeric rating scale where 1 = no distress and 5 = extensive distress
Developed through literature review and patient interviews Original language: American-English	partner and anxiety		Suitable for distribution by mail	Scores are summed and higher scores reflect more distress. Total symptom distress can be obtained as the unweighted sum of the 13 items with scores ranging from 13 to 65
Memorial Symptom Assessment Scale (MSAS) (Portenoy et al 1994)	Psychological symptoms, high-prevalence physical symptoms and low-prevalence physical symptoms	32 symptoms each assessed using three rating scales	Self-administered Verbal instructions not essential prior to administration Suitable for distribution by mail	Symptoms rated on three dimensions using 4-point rating scale to assess frequency, severity and distress

Source: Sidani 2003, Portenoy et al 1994.

The Symptom Distress Scale (McCorkle & Young 1978) was designed for use in patients with all types of cancers. One-month test–retest reliability was reported to be 0.78 in a sample of patients with lung cancer and myocardial infarction, with Cronbach's alpha internal reliability coefficients reported to be 0.83 for adults with lung cancer and 0.75 for adults with myocardial infarction (McCorkle & Benoliel 1983). Its brevity and ease of rating and scoring make it a useful tool for research. However, its focus is primarily on assessing the severity dimension of a person's symptoms.

The Memorial Symptom Assessment Scale (MSAS) (Portenoy et al 1994) is a patient-rated instrument that assesses 32 high-prevalence and low-prevalence symptoms commonly associated with cancer. Unlike most symptom assessments, this measure assesses symptoms across three dimensions: frequency; severity; and level of distress. It comprises three major symptom groups: psychological symptoms; high-prevalence physical symptoms; and low-prevalence physical symptoms. Internal consistency for the high-prevalence physical symptoms and the psychological symptoms subscales is high (Cronbach's alpha coefficient is 0.88 and 0.83 respectively), and is moderate for low-prevalence physical symptoms (Cronbach's alpha coefficient is 0.58). Summary scores and subscale scores of the MSAS correlate with well-validated measures of symptoms, quality of life, performance status and mental health ($r = 0.19$ to 0.82). It has been used with patients receiving palliative care and has been found to discriminate between patients at different stages of disease.

13.4.2 Measures of individual symptoms

This section examines commonly used instruments for measuring the symptoms of pain and fatigue.

13.4.2.1 Pain

A wide variety of measures of pain are reported in the literature. Three commonly used single-item ratings of pain intensity include numeric rating scales (a range of numbers usually 0 for no pain to 10 for highest pain, with respondents told to indicate which number best represents their pain); verbal descriptor scales (a list of descriptors that represent varying degrees of pain intensity); and visual analogue scales (a line usually 100 mm long with anchors at each end indicating extremes of pain intensity, with respondents being asked to place a mark on the line to represent his or her pain intensity) (see Table 13.2). These single-item measures are reported to be reliable and valid, although some scales appear to be easier for patients to understand and to use. Visual analogue scales (VAS) usually show higher failure rates than numeric rating scales and verbal descriptor scales. VAS measures are also identified by patients as the least preferred of the three measurement instruments (Jensen 2003). Other less commonly used single-item measures of pain intensity include a mechanical visual analogue scale, where the respondent moves a slider between the two extremes of pain on a plastic or cardboard scale, and the faces scale of pain, where drawings of facial expressions represent increasing levels of pain intensity (Jensen 2003).

Table 13.2 Single-item measures of pain

Visual analogue scales:*

Place a mark on the line below to indicate how bad you feel your pain is today:

No pain _____ Pain as bad as it could possibly be

Verbal descriptor scales:

Choose the number of the word that best describes your pain right now:

0	No pain
1	Mild
2	Moderate
3	Severe
4	Unbearable

Numeric rating scales:**

Rate your pain by circling the one number that tells how much pain you have had on average during the past week:

0	1	2	3	4	5	6	7	8	9	10
No pain										Pain as bad as you can imagine

* A 100 mm line is recommended for VAS.

** Extract from the Brief Pain Inventory (Cleeland & Ryan 1994).

Single-item measures are useful in clinical research; however, they assess a single dimension of the pain experience—pain intensity or severity. Several multi-item measures of pain have therefore been developed to better reflect the widely held view that pain is a multidimensional experience. Typically, these multidimensional measures assess intensity or severity, as well as impact or interference of pain. Some measures also assess evaluative and affective dimensions of the pain experience, such as pain relief. Examples of the more commonly used multidimensional instruments for measuring pain are included in Table 13.3.

Table 13.3 Characteristics of two instruments for assessing pain

Instrument	Dimensions examined	Length	Administration	Scoring
Brief Pain Inventory (Cleeland & Ryan 1994) Originally constructed to measure pain caused by cancer and other diseases Original language: American-English Validated across many countries and cultures	Two primary dimensions assessed: • severity • interference Individual items assess pain history; aetiology; intensity; location; quality; interference with activities	20 items (short form comprises 9 items)	Self-administered or by interview Verbal instructions not essential prior to administration Suitable for distribution by mail	No standard scoring method, although 'worst pain' can be assessed by calculating the mean of the 4 severity items, and 'interference' can be assessed by calculating the mean of the 7 interference items
Short Form McGill Pain Questionnaire (Melzack 1987) Original language: American-English Validated across many countries and cultures	Intensity Pain-rating index (sensory dimension)	2 items 11 adjectives	Self-administered or by interview Verbal instructions not essential prior to administration Suitable for distribution by mail	Pain intensity rated by: • 6-item verbal descriptor scale (present pain intensity) • 10 cm visual analogue scale Sensory dimension: each adjective scored from 0 = none to 3 = severe. Three scores are then calculated by summing the intensity rank values of all selected words: • sensory score • affective score • total score

Source: Jensen 2003, Watt-Watson 2003, McGuire et al 2004.

The Brief Pain Inventory (Cleeland & Ryan 1994) is a widely used instrument that has been validated in different clinical populations and across many countries. Studies have shown a reliable two-factor structure (intensity and interference), high internal consistency (0.78–0.97), and associations with other measures of pain intensity, and performance status (Jensen 2003, McGuire et al 2004).

The Short Form McGill Pain Questionnaire (SF–MPQ) consists of a subset of 15 descriptors from the original MPQ, and assesses the sensory and affective dimensions of the pain experience (Melzack 1987). While there are few published validation studies, those available suggest the tool has good internal consistency. However, the two subscales of this measure correlate strongly, suggesting that these subscales may be assessing a similar underlying construct (Jensen 2003, McGuire et al 2004, Watt-Watson 2003).

Instruments have also been developed to evaluate other dimensions of the pain experience, including cognitive and behavioural aspects of pain. The Barriers Questionnaire (Ward et al 1993) is one such example of a commonly used instrument that measures cognitive aspects of pain in terms of the extent to which individuals report barriers to pain management. The most recent version of the Barriers Questionnaire (BQII) (Gunnarsdottir et al 2002) comprises 27 items assessing common patient concerns about factors such as addiction, tolerance and side effects. A review of such instruments is beyond the scope of this chapter; however, it is important to note that such instruments may be especially useful in measuring the effectiveness of educational interventions (McGuire et al 2004).

In summary, there is considerable diversity in measurement instruments for assessing pain, with major differentiating factors being the dimensions assessed by each particular instrument, as well as the ease with which they can be used by patients. As such, in addition to the standard validity and reliability criteria for determining the usefulness of a research instrument, careful consideration needs to be given to the extent to which the underlying dimensions being assessed are consistent with the purpose of the investigation.

13.4.2.2 Fatigue

Like other symptoms, fatigue is conceptualised as a multidimensional experience, comprising physical, affective, cognitive and behavioural dimensions. Single-item measures of fatigue, using similar visual analogue and numeric rating scales to those used in the measurement of pain, have been reported (Sidani 2003). These single-item measures are reported to correlate well with other single-item intensity scales from instruments such as the Profile of Mood States, but are limited if an in-depth study of fatigue is required (Piper 2004).

The two most commonly used multi-item instruments to measure fatigue are presented in Table 13.4.

The Functional Assessment of Cancer Therapy—Fatigue subscale (FACT—F) was developed to assess fatigue for patients with cancer. This scale contains 13 fatigue items that measure the severity dimension of fatigue. The scale has a high level of test–retest reliability ($r = 0.90$) and internal consistency (0.93–0.95). The FACT—Fatigue scale is positively correlated with the Piper Fatigue Scale, although unlike the Piper Fatigue Scale patients do not need to be experiencing fatigue to answer questions within this scale (Yellen et al 1997).

The Piper Fatigue Scale is a commonly used scale in research into fatigue. It has become widely accepted because it purports to provide a multidimensional assessment of fatigue, and acknowledges subjective perception as being an important aspect of fatigue assessment. The original 42-item Piper Fatigue Scale was developed to measure four dimensions of fatigue proposed in her model: temporal (the timing of fatigue); sensory (emotional symptoms of fatigue); affective (emotional meaning attributed to fatigue); and intensity/severity (the impact and distress fatigue might have on activities of daily living) (Piper et al 1987). Internal consistency reliability estimates for the original scale and subscales were all above 0.80, and face and content validity were determined by a literature review and review by an 11-member national fatigue expert panel (Piper et al 1998). Concurrent validity was established by significant correlations between the subscales and mood disturbance scores of the Profile of Mood States (POMS) and the Fatigue Symptom Checklist (Piper et al 1989).

Table 13.4 Characteristics of two instruments for assessing fatigue

Instrument	Dimensions examined	Length	Administration	Scoring
Piper Fatigue Scale—Revised Original language: American-English	Temporal, affective, sensory and severity	22 items in revised scale with 3 open-ended questions 2–5 minutes to complete	Self-administered Verbal instructions not essential prior to administration Suitable for distribution by mail	Each item measured on an 11-item numeric rating scale (0–10); total fatigue and 4 subscale scores calculated, ranging between 0 and 10
Functional Assessment of Cancer Therapy—Fatigue subscale (Yellen et al 1997) Original language: American-English	Severity	13 items	Self-administered Verbal instructions not essential prior to administration Suitable for distribution by mail	Fatigue experiences rated on a 5-point Likert scale ranging from 0 = not at all to 4 = very much so

Source: Sidani 2003, Piper 2004.

More recently, Piper et al (1998) reported a study designed to reduce the total number of scale items from this original scale without decreasing the instrument's reliability. The researchers reported that this revised 22-item scale had a coherent four-factor structure, resulting in four subscales with reliabilities ranging from 0.92 to 0.97. These subscales are similar to those in the original scale and are reported to assess behavioural/severity, affective meaning, sensory and cognitive/mood dimensions of fatigue (Piper et al 1998).

13.5 The future of symptom measurement

Two potential areas for future research are the measurement of 'symptom clusters' and understanding what a particular score on a symptom measurement scale means to the individual themselves.

13.5.1 Understanding symptom clusters

A substantial body of knowledge has developed concerning the measurement of multiple and individual symptoms. However, while the presence of concurrent symptoms is generally acknowledged as a key factor influencing symptom experiences, the vast majority of research on symptom measurement so far has focused on the study of single symptoms, such as pain or fatigue. Since patients with chronic conditions commonly present with several concurrent symptoms, future advances in symptom assessment require that we develop a better understanding of the way symptoms relate to each other and the implications of these relationships for their measurement.

As such, a number of studies have emerged that have focused on understanding the underlying dimensions of symptoms, or symptom clusters, in patients with a range of conditions. For example, studies of people with cancer indicate that sleep problems, fatigue and pain often occur concurrently in patients with cancer, and that the presence of these clusters of symptoms may lead to greater morbidity (Dodd et al 2001b, Given et al 2003).

The implications of this emerging work for symptom assessment and for clinical practice are not yet well described. Dodd et al (2001a) raise a number of questions that remain unresolved as a result, such as: Is there a temporal pattern to symptom clusters? Does one symptom occur first that might be recognised as a predictor of subsequent symptoms or morbidity? Can targeting of one symptom improve outcomes for other symptoms?

13.5.2 Understanding clinical significance and individual meaning of symptoms

There is increasing interest in understanding what a particular score on a symptom measurement scale means to the individual themselves, and what implications such changes have for clinical practice. That is, if an intervention achieves a mean decrease in symptom scores of one point on a 10-point severity scale, what does this change actually mean to an individual patient? Indeed, it has become a standard requirement that research reports address the issue of statistical power, indicating what effect size and confidence intervals associated with changes in symptom scores are statistically and clinically important. The importance of determining whether a quantitative change or statistical conclusion makes a qualitative difference to a person's life is thus increasingly recognised as being integral to advancing symptom management.

Recently, a number of researchers have attempted to study these issues empirically to determine the minimum clinically significant difference required for a change symptom score to be meaningful to patients. For example, Kelly (2001) hypothesised that a clinically important change in a pain severity score was the mean difference between current and preceding scores when the person reported 'a little worse' or 'a little better' pain. Similarly, Farrar et al (2000) defined clinical importance as the proportion of patients who achieved relief in a clinical trial, as measured by whether the patient required an additional rescue medication for episodes of pain. The main point emphasised by this work is that what change is meaningful or important will depend in part on who is asked (LeFort 1993). This is especially the case in the measurement of symptoms.

13.6 Conclusion

Symptoms represent a response to disease and treatment that are a core focus for nursing activity. As such, research to develop valid and reliable measurement tools should be a key focus of nursing research. A wide range of generic and disease-specific symptom measures are available for use in research and practice. When choosing from among these instruments, consideration should be given to the strength of the psychometric properties of that instrument, as well as the applicability and feasibility of using that instrument in the population of interest. While there have been some promising developments in the field of symptom assessment, further advances may need to reflect a better understanding of the meaning of the symptom experience to individuals, and how the complex interrelationships between various personal, clinical and environmental factors influence symptom experiences.

13.7 Discussion questions

1. What are the key dimensions of a comprehensive approach to measuring symptoms?
2. What are the strengths and limitations of instruments that measure: (a) single dimensions of a symptom; and (b) multiple dimensions of a symptom?
3. What factors should be taken into account when selecting an instrument for measuring symptoms?
4. A patient's mean pain score on a numeric rating scale ranging from 0 (no pain) to 10 (pain as bad as it could be) reduces from 4.2 to 3.5. Discuss how we might consider the clinical significance of this reduction in mean score.
5. How useful are the instruments described in this chapter for a patient who is cognitively impaired? Provide reasons for your answers.

13.8 References

Aaronson N, Ahmedzai S, Bergman B et al 1993 The European Organization for Research and Treatment of Cancer QLQ–30: A quality of life instrument for use in international clinical trials in oncology. *Journal of the National Cancer Institute* 85:365–76.

Blyth F M, March L M, Brnabic A J et al 2001 Chronic pain in Australia: a prevalence study. *Pain* 89(2–3):127–34.

Bowling A 1995 *Measuring disease*. Open University Press, Buckingham.

Caroci Ade S, Lareau S C 2004 Descriptors of dyspnea by patients with chronic obstructive pulmonary disease versus congestive heart failure. *Heart & Lung: The Journal of Critical Care* 33(2):102–10.

Cleeland C, Ryan K 1994 Pain assessment. Global use of the Brief Pain Inventory. *Annals Academy Medicine* 23:129–38.

Corner J, Bailey C (eds) 2001 *Cancer nursing: care in context*, p 336. Blackwell, Oxford.

Dodd M, Janson S, Facione N et al 2001a Advancing the science of symptom management. *Journal of Advanced Nursing* 33(5):668–76.

Dodd M, Miaskowski C, Paul S 2001b Symptom clusters and their effect on the functional status of patients with cancer. *Oncology Nursing Forum* 28(3):465–70.

Doran D 2003 *Nursing-sensitive outcomes: state of the science*. Jones & Bartlett, Sudbury.

Farrar J L, Portenoy R K, Berlin J A et al 2000 Defining clinically important difference in pain outcome measures. *Pain* 88:287–94.

Frank-Stromborg M, Olsen S (eds) 2004 *Instruments for clinical health care research*, 3rd edn. Jones & Bartlett, Sudbury.

Gift A G, Stommel M, Jablonski A, Given W 2003 A cluster of symptoms over time in patients with lung cancer. *Nursing Research* 52(6):393–400.

Given C, Given B, Azzouz F et al 2001 Predictors of pain and fatigue in the year following diagnosis among elderly cancer patients. *Journal of Pain and Symptom Management* 21(6):456–66.

Gunnarsdottir S, Donovan H, Serlin R 2002 Patient-related barriers to pain management: The barriers questionnaire II (BQII). *Pain* 99:385–96.

Jensen M 2003 The validity and reliability of pain measures in adults with cancer. *Journal of Pain* 4(1):2–21.

Kelly A 2001 The minimum clinically significant difference in visual analogue scale pain score does not differ with pain severity. *Emergency Medicine Journal* 18(3):205–7.

Keogh E, Herdenfeldt M 2002 Gender, coping and the perception of pain. *Pain* 97(3):195–201.

LeFort S M 1993 The statistical versus clinical significance debate. *Image: Journal of Nursing Scholarship* 25(1):57–62.

McCaffery M, Pasero C 1999 Underlying complexities, misconceptions and practical tools, in M McCaffery & C Pasero, *Pain Clinical Manual*, pp 35–99. Mosby, St Louis.

McCorkle R, Benoliel J 1983 Symptom distress, current concerns and mood disturbance after diagnosis of life-threatening disease. *Social Science and Medicine* 17:431–8.

McCorkle R, Young K 1978 Development of a symptom distress scale. *Cancer Nursing* 5:373–8.

McGuire D, Kim H, Lang X 2004 Measuring pain, in M Frank-Stromborg & S J Olsen (eds) *Instruments for clinical health care research.* Jones & Bartlett, Sudbury.

McPherson C J, Addington-Hall J M 2003 Judging the quality of care at the end of life: can proxies provide reliable information? *Social Science and Medicine* 56(1):95–109.

Melzack R 1987 The short-form McGill Pain Questionnaire. *Pain* 30:191–7.

Mercadante S, Cassucio A, Fulfaro F 2000 The course of symptom frequency and intensity in advanced cancer patients followed at home. *Journal of Pain and Symptom Management* 20(2):104–12.

Nekolaichuk C L, Maguire T O, Suarez-Almazor M et al 1999 Assessing the reliability of patient, nurse and family caregiver symptom ratings in hospitalized advanced cancer patients. *Journal of Clinical Oncology* 17(11):3621–30.

Piper B 2004 Measuring fatigue, in M Frank-Stromborg and S Olsen (eds) 2004 *Instruments for clinical health care research*, 3rd edn, pp 538–69. Jones & Bartlett, Sudbury.

Piper B F, Dibble S L, Dodd M J et al 1998 The Revised Piper Fatigue Scale: psychometric evaluation in women with breast cancer. *Oncology Nursing Forum* 25(4):677–84.

Piper B, Dodd M, Paul S, Weleer S 1989 The development of an instrument to measure the subjective dimension of fatigue, in S Funk, M Tornquist & L Champagne et al (eds) *Key aspects of comfort management of pain, fatigue and nausea.* Springer, New York.

Piper B, Lindsey A, Dodd M 1987 Fatigue mechanisms in cancer patients: developing nursing theory. *Oncology Nursing Forum* 14(6):17–23.

Pleym H, Spigset O, Kharasch E D, Dale O 2003 Gender differences in drug effects: implications for anesthesiologists. *Acta Anaesthesiologica Scandinavica* 47(3):241–59.

Portenoy R, Thaler H, Kornblith A et al 1994 The Memorial Symptom Assessment Scale: an instrument for the evaluation of symptom prevalence, characteristics, and distress. *European Journal of Cancer* 30A:1226–36.

Pringle D, Doran D 2003 Patient outcomes as an accountability, in D Doran (ed) *Nursing-sensitive outcomes: state of the science.* Jones & Bartlett, Sudbury.

Schwartz A L, Nail L M, Chen S et al 2000 Fatigue patterns observed in patients receiving chemotherapy and radiotherapy. *Cancer Investigation* 18(1):11–19.

Sidani S 2003 Symptom management, in D Doran (ed) *Nursing-sensitive outcomes: state of the science*. Jones & Bartlett, Sudbury.

Smith M, Stullenbarger E 1995 An integrative review and meta-analysis of oncology nursing research: 1981–1990. *Cancer Nursing* 18(3):167–79.

Sutcliffe-Chidgey J, Holmes S 1996 Developing a symptom distress scale for terminal malignant disease. *International Journal of Palliative Nursing* 2:496–511.

Ward S, Goldberg N, Miller-McCauley V et al Patient-related barriers to management of cancer pain. *Pain* 52:319–24.

Ware J, Sherbourne C 1992 The MOS 36-item short form health survey (SF–36): I. Conceptual framework and item selection. *Medical Care* 30:473–83.

Watt-Watson J 2003 Pain as a symptom outcome, in D Doran (ed) *Nursing-sensitive outcomes: state of the science*. Jones & Bartlett, Sudbury.

Yellen S B, Cella D, Webster K et al 1997 Measuring fatigue and other anemia-related symptoms with the Functional Assessment of Cancer Therapy (FACT) Measurement System. *Journal of Pain and Symptom Management* 13(2):63–74.

chapter 14

Instruments to measure health-related quality of life as a nursing outcome

Jan McDowell and Helen Edwards

14.1 Learning objectives

After reading this chapter, you should be able to:

1. *describe the concept of health-related quality of life*
2. *describe the importance of measuring health-related quality of life*
3. *differentiate between general and specific measures of health-related quality of life, and*
4. *analyse how different measures of health-related quality of life influence the evidence obtained when conducting nursing research.*

14.2 Introduction

The purpose of this chapter is to provide an overview of instruments designed to measure aspects of health-related quality of life (HRQOL), an outcome of interest to an increasing number of nurse researchers. This is because many interventions undertaken by nurses are aimed at improving quality of life (QOL) for patients. In an outcome-focused and evidenced-based practice (EBP) context, nurses are required to demonstrate that nursing interventions do achieve expected outcomes. To do this, nurses need to be able to measure the outcomes of care, in this case, QOL.

QOL is a nebulous concept that has been discussed for thousands of years. Definitions are diverse and vary across disciplines. Greek philosophers associated QOL with 'happiness'. Since that time others have broadly described QOL as 'goodness', 'fulfilment' or 'wellbeing' (Bowling 1997, Haas 1999). Many illnesses and conditions can impact on a person's sense of fulfilment and wellbeing; hence the interest in HRQOL by nurses. Evidence derived from investigations of patients' HRQOL is used by scientists, clinicians and politicians to guide patient management and health-related policy decision-making (Bowling 1995).

The chapter begins with a general discussion about measuring QOL, followed by a more focused discussion on measuring HRQOL. The remainder of the chapter discusses the measurement of specific aspects of HRQOL. Details of relevant instruments are also outlined.

14.3 What is health-related quality of life?

At the broadest level, the quality of a person's life encompasses physical, emotional, psychological, spiritual, recreational and economic aspects. From a biopsychosocial perspective, QOL has been defined as 'a concept encompassing a broad range of physical and psychological characteristics and limitations which describe an individual's ability to function and derive satisfaction from so doing' (Walker & Rosser 1993:383). Essentially this statement describes physical, social and emotional wellbeing—constructs that are now considered to be key elements of HRQOL.

Understanding QOL in terms of health is not a recent phenomenon. For instance, objective indicators of HRQOL such as mortality, hospital readmissions, recurrence of health events, and return to work have been examined for decades (Bowling 1995). During the 1970s there was a growing awareness among health researchers that the concept of HRQOL encompassed more than the incidence of major morbidity or mortality (Salek 1998). The realisation that assisting patients to have a 'comfortable, functional, and satisfying life-style' (Salek 1998:1) was important when a disease condition could not be cured and began a surge of interest in evaluating patients' own perceptions of their health status and wellbeing (Guyatt & Cook 1994). This interest has increased markedly since that time, particularly during the past decade.

Nurses are also interested in exploring the impact of acute and chronic conditions on patients' HRQOL. Examples of recent studies that inform nursing practice include:

- examining the relationship between insomnia and HRQOL in patients with chronic illness (Katz & McHorney 2002)
- investigating the impact of fatigue on HRQOL in patients with advanced cancer (Knobel et al 2003)
- comparing HRQOL between two groups of cancer patients (Bostrom et al 2003), and
- exploring how different models of chronic disease management affect patients' HRQOL (Litaker et al 2003).

Despite the ever-increasing body of literature about HRQOL, there continues to be confusion as to the definition of the construct. One definition of HRQOL is 'the value assigned to duration of life as modified by the impairments, functional states, perceptions, and social opportunities that are influenced by disease, injury, treatment, or policy' (Patrick & Erickson 1993:20). Bowling (1997:6) defines HRQOL as 'individual responses to the physical, mental and social effects of illness on daily living which influence the extent to which personal satisfaction with life circumstances can be achieved'. There are many other definitions of HRQOL, and a range of examples can be found in a comprehensive guide to HRQOL measurement published by Salek (1998).

The interchangeable use of the terms 'HRQOL' and 'health status' in HRQOL literature creates further confusion. Salek (1998) attributes this to a lack of operational definitions for the two concepts. Dijkers (1999) and Guyatt et al (1993) ascribe it to differing views between disciplines within a multidisciplinary field of health-related research (e.g. social versus medical scientists). Salek (1998:3) attempts to differentiate between the concepts by defining health status as 'a measure of an individual's function in terms of physical, social and mental well-being', and HRQOL as the 'level of an individual's total well-being and satisfaction with life and how this is affected by disease and treatment'. Collectively, these two definitions appear to be little different from the definition proposed by Bowling (1997) that is presented in the previous paragraph.

Despite the ongoing debate about a definitive explanation of the concept, researchers generally view HRQOL as a multidimensional construct that includes physical and emotional wellbeing. Many researchers also include social wellbeing in the construct (Bowling 1997, Dijkers 1999, Haas 1999, Oldridge 1997, Salek 1998). Indeed, there is evidence to suggest that social wellbeing may not be a separate dimension, as it is highly correlated with emotional wellbeing (Lim et al 1998, Ware et al 1994). Therefore, in the absence of a universally accepted definition for HRQOL, and in the interests of parsimony in this chapter, any reference to general HRQOL will be describing physical and emotional wellbeing with the assumption that emotional wellbeing also includes social wellbeing.

HRQOL research has gained considerable momentum during the past decade as investigators recognise that patients' self-assessment of their health is a better predictor of patients' wellbeing than clinical indicators (Guyatt et al 1993). Nursing outcomes research is increasingly centred on self-assessed measures of wellbeing. For example, an online search of the CINAHL database using the term 'health-related quality of life' revealed that 113 articles were published in nursing journals between 1992 and 2004. Ninety-six (85%) of these articles have been published since 2000.

14.4 Instruments for measuring health-related quality of life

During the past three decades many different instruments have been developed to assess HRQOL. Sanders et al (1998) provided some indication of the number when they analysed the reporting of 'quality of life' in 67 published randomised controlled trials and found that 48 of the studies used 62 different established instruments, and another 15 studies used newly developed instruments. The majority of these instruments measured health-related aspects of QOL. Gill and Feinstein (1994) also analysed the reporting of 'quality of life' in a review of 75 scientific papers published in medical literature. The authors determined that a total of 159 instruments were used in the studies, and, of these, 136 were only used once. Again, the majority of identified instruments in the Gill and Feinstein (1994) review measured health-related aspects of QOL. Thus, a wide variety of instruments is available and the task of choosing an appropriate instrument for a research project is not an easy one.

Most of the better known and more widely used instruments can be loosely categorised as generic or condition-specific measures of HRQOL. Another category comprises instruments that measure individual aspects of HRQOL. *Generic* instruments are designed to be used with a wide range of patient and population samples. *Condition-specific* measures are deliberately narrow in focus and useful with patients who have a particular illness or symptom (e.g. cardiac disease, angina or depression). The third category of HRQOL instruments measures *specific or individual aspects*, such as social support or functional status.

14.4.1 Generic instruments

Generic measures of HRQOL tend to be grouped according to whether they are utility indices or health profiles. Utility indices are generally calculated by economists using cost–unit analyses and are expressed in terms of quality-adjusted life years (QALY). One method of calculating QALY is to multiply the average number of additional years of life gained from a medical intervention by a judgment of the patients' QOL in each of those years. The outcome is a single weighted score (Salek 1998).

In contrast, outcomes from health profiles provide a multifaceted perspective of a person's HRQOL, as scores can be calculated for different dimensions and presented separately, or as an aggregated global score. Health profiles are useful for large studies such as national health surveys, as they provide snapshots of population HRQOL. Health profiles are also popular with researchers and clinicians who are interested in obtaining a broader perspective of the effect of disease on a person's wellbeing by comparing the outcomes with those of a normal population (Bowling 1997, Mayou & Bryant 1993, Salek 1998). Health profile instruments can vary in the constructs that they measure but the common goal is to capture HRQOL 'as perceived by the patient in areas of health identified to be of value to the patient' (Rumsfeld et al 1999:2).

State-of-the-art literature reviews have identified four generic measures of HRQOL that are commonly used in health research (Bowling 1997, Dempster & Donnelly 2000, Fletcher et al 1992, McDowell & Newell 1996, Patrick & Erickson 1993, Sanders et al 1998). These four instruments are:
• the Nottingham Health Profile (Hunt et al 1986)
• the Sickness Impact Profile (Bergner et al 1976)
• the McMaster Health Index Questionnaire (Chambers et al 1976), and
• the Medical Outcomes Study (MOS) Short Form 36 (Ware et al 1993).
The characteristics of the four instruments are summarised in Table 14.1.

Table 14.1 Characteristics of four *generic* measures of health-related quality of life

Instrument	Dimensions examined	Length	Administration	Scoring
Nottingham Health Profile (NHP) (Hunt et al 1981)	Part I—6 dimensions of experience: pain; physical mobility; sleep; emotional reactions; energy; social isolation	45 items	Self or interviewer (10–15 minutes) Verbal instructions not essential prior to administration	Weighted scores for: 6 dimensions 7 single items
Developed in UK from interviews with ill and healthy laypeople	Part II—7 dimensions of daily life: employment; household work; relationships; personal		Suitable for distribution by mail	Possible scores: 0 = best 100 = worst
Original language: English	life; sex; hobbies; vacations			

(continued)

Instrument	Dimensions examined	Length	Administration	Scoring
Sickness Impact Profile (SIP) (Bergner et al 1976) Developed in US from literature and interviews with health professionals, ill and healthy laypeople Original language: American-English	Physical: ambulation; mobility; body care and movement Psychosocial: communication; alertness; emotional behaviour; social interaction Other: sleep and rest; eating; work; home management; recreational pastimes	136 items	Self or interviewer (30–50 minutes) Verbal instructions required prior to administration Not recommended for distribution by mail	Weighted scores for: 12 dimensions 2 summaries (physical and psychosocial functioning) 1 overall profile Possible scores: 0 = best 100 = worst
McMaster Health Index Questionnaire (MHIQ) (Chambers et al 1976) Developed in Canada from literature; interviews with health professionals and 'brainstorming' among authors Original language: English; Canadian-French	Physical: mobility; self-care activities; communication Social: general wellbeing; work/social role performance/material welfare; social support Emotional: self-esteem; personal relationships; expectations of future; critical life events	59 items	Self or interviewer (20 minutes) Verbal instructions not essential prior to administration Suitable for distribution by mail	Standardised scores for: 3 summaries (physical, social and emotional functioning) Possible scores: 0 = worst 1 = best
Medical Outcomes Study Short Form 36 (SF–36) (Ware et al 1993) Developed in US from other health assessment instruments Original language: American-English	8 dimensions: physical functioning; role limitations due to physical problems; bodily pain; general health; vitality; social functioning; role limitations due to emotional problems; mental health Other: change in health state	36 items	Self or interviewer (10–15 minutes) Verbal instructions not essential prior to administration Suitable for distribution by mail	Recoded (if necessary) and transformed scores: 8 dimensions Weighted scores: 2 summaries (physical and mental) Possible scores: 0 = worst 100 = best

Source: Bowling 1997, McDowell & Newell 1996, Salek 1998, Walker & Rosser 1993, Ware et al 1993, Wenger et al 1984.

14.4.1.1 Nottingham Health Profile

The first of the instruments, the Nottingham Health Profile (NHP), is used in clinical trials and population surveys, as well as in the clinical setting (Hunt et al 1981, McDowell & Newell 1996). The instrument, consisting of two parts, comprises 45 items with response options of 'yes' or 'no'. The first part (38 items) assesses six experiential dimensions of HRQOL, whereas the second part measures seven dimensions of activities of daily life. The specific dimensions for each part of the instrument are listed in Table 14.1. This instrument is widely used to assess HRQOL and is reported to be psycho-metrically valid and reliable in general populations (Bowling 1997, Dempster & Donnelly 2000, Sanders et al 1998).

14.4.1.2 Sickness Impact Profile

The Sickness Impact Profile (SIP) is designed to detect change in health status over time, or differences between groups. It is also used as an outcome meas-ure when evaluating health delivery services (Bergner et al 1976, 1981). The SIP comprises 136 items that measure two dimensions of HRQOL (i.e. physi-cal and psychosocial), plus a number of other factors that are listed in Table 14.1. Responses are 'yes' if a particular item is relevant to them on a given day (e.g. 'I sit during much of the day') (Bowling 1997:40). If a particular item is not relevant to the participant, then that item is not answered. Some researchers have criticised the structures of the NHP and the SIP, and argue that these instruments measure the effects of illness on specific behaviours, rather than global HRQOL (Bowling 1997, McDowell & Newell 1996). Psychometric evidence from studies of patients appears to be satisfactory (Dempster & Donnelly 2000).

14.4.1.3 McMaster Health Index Questionnaire

The McMaster Health Index Questionnaire (MHIQ) was developed for use in clinical research primarily with outpatients living in the community. It has also been used for evaluating health services. The MHIQ comprises 59 items that measure three dimensions of HRQOL: physical, social and emotional wellbeing. Further details of these dimensions are provided in Table 14.1. Response options are a mix of dichotomous (yes/no), and five-point Likert-type scales (strongly agree–strongly disagree; good–poor). The instrument is reported as having acceptable psychometric properties in general popula-tions (Bowling 1997, Chambers et al 1976, McDowell & Newell 1996, Wenger et al 1984).

14.4.1.4 Medical Outcomes Study Short Form 36 (SF–36)

The Medical Outcomes Study Short Form 36 (SF–36), originally developed to measure population health status, is the most recent of the four instruments. It is a well-known generic measure of HRQOL that is widely used to evalu-ate the progression of chronic disease, and the effectiveness of treatment interventions (Dempster & Donnelly 2000, Ware & Sherbourne 1992). The SF–36 comprises 35 items grouped into eight scales that collectively measure dimensions of physical and emotional wellbeing, and one item that meas-ures change in health status over time. Response options for the majority of items are ordinal (Ware et al 1993). The psychometric properties of the instrument are reported to be good (Dempster & Donnelly 2000, McDowell & Newell 1996).

14.4.2 Condition-specific instruments

Health researchers who use condition-specific instruments to measure HRQOL prefer to do so because the instruments are designed to assess life issues that tend to be affected by a particular disease or symptom. Other reasons for using them are that the contents are relevant to participants (Dijkers 1999), and the outcomes are interpretable by clinicians (Oldridge

1997). Many condition-specific instruments exist. Therefore, we have chosen to focus on instruments designed to be used with people who have cardiac disease or depression, as the prevalence of these conditions in the community is high.

Two *disease-specific* measures of HRQOL that are commonly used in cardiac-related research are the Quality of Life after Acute Myocardial Infarction Questionnaire (QLMI) (Oldridge et al 1991) and the Quality of Life Index—Cardiac Version III (QLI) (Faris & Stotts 1990, Ferrans & Powers 1985). The characteristics of the two instruments are summarised in Table 14.2. Two *symptom-specific* measures of HRQOL are the Seattle Angina Questionnaire (SAQ) (Spertus et al 1995) and the Edinburgh Postpartum Depression Scale (EPDS) (Cox et al 1987). The characteristics of these instruments are summarised in Table 14.3.

Table 14.2 Characteristics of two *disease-specific* measures of health-related quality of life

Instrument	Dimensions examined	Length	Administration	Scoring
Quality of Life after Acute Myocardial Infarction (QLMI) (Oldridge et al 1991) Developed in US from interviews with health professionals with experience in cardiac rehabilitation, post-AMI patients and literature reviews Original language: American-English	Physical limitations: symptoms; restrictions Emotions: confidence; self-esteem; emotion	26 items	Self or interviewer (10 minutes) Verbal instructions not essential prior to administration Suitable for distribution by mail	Dimension scores: Average of responses to items in each dimension Global score: Average of responses to all 26 items Possible scores: 1 = worst 7 = best
Quality of Life Index—Cardiac Version III (QLI) (Ferrans & Powers 1984) Developed in US from literature and interviews with patients Original language: American-English	Part I (36 items): satisfaction with health and functioning; socioeconomic; psychological/spiritual; family areas of life Part II (36 items): importance of health and functioning; socioeconomic; psychological/spiritual; family areas of life	72 items	Self (15 minutes) Verbal instructions not essential prior to administration Suitable for distribution by mail	Weighted scores for: 4 dimensions Part I scores are weighted by the responses on Part II Possible scores: 0 = worst 30 = best

Source: Bowling 1997, Ferrans & Powers 1985, McDowell & Newell 1996, Oldridge et al 1991, Salek 1998.

14.4.2.1 Quality of Life after Acute Myocardial Infarction Questionnaire

The Quality of Life after Acute Myocardial Infarction Questionnaire (QLMI) was initially developed to evaluate the effectiveness of a cardiac rehabilitation program in improving moderately anxious/depressed post-AMI patients'

HRQOL. The instrument comprises 26 items that assess a participant's perception of his or her HRQOL over the previous two weeks, and responses are rated on a seven-point Likert-type scale. Factor analyses demonstrate that the instrument measures two (i.e. limitations and emotions) (Oldridge et al 1991) or three (i.e. physical, social and emotional) (Heller et al 1993) dimensions of HRQOL. The measure was originally designed to be administered by a trained interviewer (Oldridge et al 1991), but has since been adapted for use as a self-administered questionnaire (Heller et al 1993, Lim et al 1993). The QLMI is a valid and reliable instrument that is able to discriminate between patient groups and evaluate changes in HRQOL over time (Hillers et al 1994, Oldridge et al 1998).

A modified version, the QLMI–2 (also known as the MacNew), is one that was adapted for use with Australian patients. It comprises 27 items and the outcomes are presented as dimension scores and/or a global score of HRQOL (Dixon et al 2002, Lim et al 1998). The self-administered instrument demonstrates strong internal consistency with Cronbach's alpha coefficients exceeding 0.90 for the three dimensions (Valenti et al 1996), and is reported as having adequate discriminant validity in studies of post-AMI patients (Dempster & Donnelly 2000).

14.4.2.2 Quality of Life Index—Cardiac Version III
The Quality of Life Index (QLI) was developed for use with dialysis patients (Ferrans & Powers 1985) and adapted for use with cardiac patients (Faris & Stotts 1990). The instrument measures four dimensions of HRQOL: health and functioning; socioeconomic; psychosocial/spiritual; and family (Dempster & Donnelly 2000). There are two parts to the measure: Part I asks participants to rate the importance of 36 items, and Part II seeks patients' level of satisfaction with the same 36 items. The QLI is reported as being a reliable instrument with test–retest correlations ranging from 0.70–0.90, and Cronbach's alpha coefficients of 0.90 or greater in samples of cardiac patients (Bowling 1995, Dempster & Donnelly 2000). It has also demonstrated responsiveness over time (Faris & Stotts 1990).

14.4.2.3 Seattle Angina Questionnaire
The Seattle Angina Questionnaire (SAQ) was developed to assess the physical and emotional effects of angina. Five clinically important domains of HRQOL are measured with 19 items, and responses are rated on five-item or six-item Likert-type scales. The dimensions measured over the previous four weeks are physical limitations (9 items), anginal stability (1 item), anginal frequency (2 items), treatment satisfaction (4 items) and disease perception (3 items) (Dempster & Donnelly 2000, Spertus et al 1995). Psychometric testing of the instrument has been undertaken and most of the dimensions are reported to be valid, reliable and sensitive to clinical change. However, the responsive estimate for the treatment satisfaction dimension and the test–retest reliability estimates for the anginal stability dimension, based on reported mean three-month changes in cardiac patients, are low (Spertus et al 1995), suggesting that these particular subscales may not be useful as evaluative measures (Dempster & Donnelly 2000).

Table 14.3 Characteristics of two *symptom-specific* measures of health-related quality of life

Instrument	Dimensions examined	Length	Administration	Scoring
Seattle Angina Questionnaire (SAQ) (Spertus et al 1995) Developed in US from literature, existing instruments and interviews with clinicians Original language: American-English	Physical limitations Anginal stability Anginal frequency Treatment satisfaction Disease perception	19 items	Self (time to administer not reported) Verbal instructions not essential prior to administration Suitable for distribution by mail	Transformed scores for: 5 dimensions Possible scores: 0 = worst 100 = best
Edinburgh Postpartum Depression Scale (EPDS) (Cox et al 1987) Developed at Health Centres in the United Kingdom Original language: UK-English	Anxiety Insomnia Sadness Self-blame Self-harm	10 items	Self (5 minutes) Verbal instructions not essential prior to administration Suitable for distribution by mail	Global score calculated by summing responses Possible scores: 0 = best 30 = worst

Source: Bowling 1997, Cox et al 1987, Davis et al 2003, Spertus et al 1995.

14.4.2.4 Edinburgh Postpartum Depression Scale

The Edinburgh Postpartum Depression Scale (EPDS) was developed as a screening tool for assessing depressive symptomatology in women following childbirth. Five important domains of depression are measured with 10 items, and responses are rated on a four-point Likert-type scale ranging from 0–3 (Cox et al 1987, Davis et al 2003). The dimensions measured over the previous week are anxiety (2 items), insomnia (1 item), sadness (5 items), self-blame (1 item) and self-harm (1 item). Seven of the items are reverse-scored prior to summing the 10 responses to achieve a global score (Cox et al 1987). Psychometric testing of the instrument has been widely undertaken and the instrument is reported to be valid, reliable and sensitive to clinical change (Sharp & Lipsky 2002).

14.4.3 Instruments for individual aspects

In some care contexts, using instruments that measure individual aspects of HRQOL may be more useful than using generic or condition-specific measures. Health researchers, who are interested in investigating the impact of a condition or intervention on a particular aspect of HRQOL, may prefer to use an instrument that is designed to collect specific information about that aspect. Many nursing interventions are targeted at specific aspects of care and are offered over a relatively short period of time. Therefore, nurses often choose to focus on a relevant element of HRQOL as an outcome for their research rather than measure HRQOL at the broader level.

Of the many instruments that are available to assess individual aspects of HRQOL, measures of social support and functional status are profiled, as they are outcomes that are commonly used in nursing research. The selected instruments are the Arizona Social Support Interview Schedule (ASSIS) (Barrera 1981), and the Total Activities of Daily Living Scale (TADLS) (Zarit et al 1999). These instruments are appropriate for use with diverse groups in health research. For example, the ASSIS has been used to examine: social support for people with schizophrenia (Clinton et al 1998); AIDS-related family functioning (Murphy et al 2002); and change in social support over time for chronically impaired older adults (Reinhardt et al 2003). The TADLS has been used to measure the functional status of primary caregivers for people with Alzheimer's disease (Wright et al 2001), depressed elderly people (Zarit et al 1999) and older care receivers (Edwards & Noller 1998). The characteristics of the two instruments are summarised in Table 14.4.

Table 14.4 Characteristics of two instruments that measure *individual aspects* of health-related quality of life

Instrument	Dimensions examined	Length	Administration	Scoring
Arizona Social Support Interview Schedule (ASSIS) (Barrera 1981)	Perceived available support: intimate interaction; material aid; guidance; feedback; physical assistance; social participation	Difficult to quantify number of items— depends upon participant responses	Structured interview (15–20 minutes)	Dimension scores: total of responses to items in each dimension
Developed in the US from literature, existing instruments and interviews with clinicians	Actual received support: intimate interaction; material aid; guidance; feedback; physical assistance; social participation			Possible scores: not applicable
	Satisfaction with received support			
	Type of support: family; friend			
Original language: American-English	Most supportive person in network			
Total Activities of Daily Living Scale (TADLS) (Zarit et al 1999)	Personal activities of daily living (8 items): getting out of bed; bathing/showering; washing self; grooming; dressing; getting to toilet; toileting; eating	16 items	Self or interviewer (15 minutes)	Dimension scores: total of responses to items in each dimension
Developed in the US from standardised assessments			Suitable for distribution by mail	Global score: total of responses to all 16 items
Original language: American-English	Instrumental activities of daily living (8 items): heavy household work; laundry; bed making; cooking; shopping; lifting or moving items; banking; telephoning			Possible global score: 16 = worst 64 = best

Source: Barrera 1981, Bowling 1997, Zarit et al 1999.

14.4.3.1 Arizona Social Support Interview Schedule

The Arizona Social Support Interview Schedule (ASSIS) is designed to collect information related to provision of social support and satisfaction with that support within an individual's social network. Affective (intimate interaction, guidance, positive feedback) and instrumental (material aid, physical assistance, social participation) dimensions of support are assessed. The ASSIS is administered as a structured interview during which participants are asked to identify individuals: (a) perceived as being available to provide support in each of the dimensions; and (b) who actually provided support in each of the dimensions during the previous month. A 'perceived available' social support score and an 'actual' social support score are calculated by totalling the number of identified individuals for available and actual support, respectively.

Demographic information (e.g. age, gender, relationship to the participant) about each identified person is also collected. These data are used to differentiate the types of support within the network (e.g. family, friend). Participants rate their satisfaction with received support on a three-point scale for each dimension. An overall 'satisfaction with support' score is calculated by summing the responses. A higher score indicates greater satisfaction. Participants also nominate the person in their network who is most supportive. Reported alpha coefficients for the ASSIS ('available network' range 0.87–0.88, 'actual network' range 0.81–0.82, 'satisfaction with support' range 0.55–0.70) indicate that the instrument is internally reliable (McDowell 1995, Slavin & Compas 1989) and stable over time, with a test–retest correlation coefficient of 0.88 over a period of two or more days (Barrera 1981).

14.4.3.2 Total Activities of Daily Living Scale

The Total Activities of Daily Living Scale (TADLS) was developed for use with the elderly and consists of 16 items drawn from widely used standardised assessments (Katz et al 1963, Lawton 1971). Two subscales measure perceived performance when undertaking eight personal (PADL) and eight instrumental (IADL) activities of daily living. Participants indicate the degree to which they believe they can perform each of these activities (e.g. shopping, bathing) on a four-point Likert-type scale. The specific activities are detailed in Table 14.4. Reported alpha coefficients indicate that the internal reliability of the two subscales is high (PADL = 0.95, IADL = 0.93) (Zarit et al 1999). The responses to both subscales are summed to create a TADL score. A higher score indicates better functional status.

14.5 Conclusion

There is continuing debate as to whether a generic or condition-specific instrument is the better measure to assess HRQOL as a nursing outcome, and advantages and disadvantages of use have been identified for both types of instruments in this chapter. As noted earlier, researchers who favour generic HRQOL instruments argue that the main advantage associated with using these measures is the opportunity to compare patient outcomes irrespective of the underlying disease condition. A further advantage is that researchers can compare patient outcomes with population norms. It has been noted that generic instruments may not be as sensitive to clinical change as disease-specific measures. However, recently published evidence suggests that the subscales of a generic measure of HRQOL (i.e. SF–36) are as sensitive as, and in some instances more sensitive than, disease-specific instruments in detecting small clinical differences in cardiac patients (Smith et al 2000).

Proponents of condition-specific measures argue that the content and outcomes are more relevant to patients and clinicians than those of generic instruments. Moreover, it is suggested that these instruments tend to be more responsive or sensitive than generic instruments to minimal changes in a particular disease condition, although this has been challenged in a recent small study of cardiac patients (Smith et al 2000). A disadvantage in using a condition-specific instrument is that outcomes from these measures can only be compared with those from other patients with the same condition.

A number of researchers suggest that using generic, condition-specific and other measures concurrently provides a better overall assessment of a patient's HRQOL (Bowling 1997, Dempster & Donnelly 2000, Salek 1998). However, the use of a number of instruments may increase respondent burden due to being asked to complete a battery of questionnaires. Participants may choose, in this scenario, to withdraw from a study, which could bias the outcomes. Thus, it is perhaps more appropriate for a nurse researcher proposing to investigate HRQOL to give due consideration to the *purpose* of the study at the outset and select an instrument that will best provide answers to specific research questions.

14.6 Discussion questions

1. What are the limitations of using instruments to measure HRQOL?
2. Would measuring HRQOL improve your nursing practice? If so, how?
3. Which type of HRQOL measure (i.e. generic/disease/symptom/other) would be most appropriate for your practice?
4. How could you use HRQOL data in your practice as a nurse?

14.7 References

Barrera M 1981 Social support in the adjustment of pregnant adolescents: assessment issues, in B H Gottlieb (ed), *Social networks and social support*, pp 69–96. Sage Publications, Beverly Hills, California.

Bergner M, Bobbitt R A, Carter W B, Gilson B S 1981 The Sickness Impact Profile: development and final revision of a health status measure. *Medical Care* 29:787–805.

Bergner M, Bobbitt R A, Pollard W E et al 1976 The Sickness Impact Profile: validation of a health status measure. *Medical Care* 14:57–67.

Bostrom B, Sandh M, Lundberg D, Fridlund B 2003 A comparison of pain and health-related quality of life between two groups of cancer patients with differing average levels of pain. *Journal of Clinical Nursing* 12(5):726–36.

Bowling A 1995 *Measuring disease: a review of disease-specific quality of life measurement scales*. Open University Press, Buckingham.

Bowling A 1997 *Measuring health: a review of quality of life measurement scales*, 2nd edn. Open University Press, Philadelphia.

Chambers L W, Sackett D L, Goldsmith C H et al 1976 Development and application of an index of social function. *Health Services Research* 11(4):430–41.

Clinton M, Lunney P, Edwards H et al 1998 Perceived social support and community adaptation in schizophrenia. *Journal of Advanced Nursing* 27(5):955–66.

Cox J L, Holden J M, Sagovsky R 1987, Detection of postnatal depression. Development of the 10-item Edinburgh Postnatal Depression Scale. *British Journal of Psychiatry* 150:782–6.

Davis L, Edwards H, Mohay H, Wollin J 2003 The course of depression in mothers of premature infants in hospital and at home. *Australian Journal of Advanced Nursing* 21(2):20–6.

Dempster M, Donnelly M 2000 Measuring the health related quality of life of people with ischaemic heart disease. *Heart* 83(6):641–4.

Dijkers M 1999 Measuring quality of life: methodological issues. *American Journal of Physical Medicine & Rehabilitation* 78(3):286–300.

Dixon T, Lim L L, Oldridge N B 2002 The MacNew heart disease health-related quality of life instrument: reference data for users. *Quality of Life Research* 11(2):173–83.

Edwards H, Noller P 1998 Factors influencing caregiver–care receiver communication and its impact on the well-being of older care receivers. *Health Communication* 10(4):317–41.

Faris J, Stotts N 1990 The effect of percutaneous transluminal coronary angioplasty on quality of life. *Progress in Cardiovascular Nursing* 5:132–40.

Ferrans C E, Powers M J 1985 Quality of Life Index: development and psychometric properties. *Advances in Nursing Science* 8:15–24.

Fletcher A, Gore S, Jones D et al 1992 Quality of life measures in health care: II. Design, analysis, and interpretation. *British Medical Journal* 305:1145–8.

Gill T M, Feinstein A R 1994 A critical appraisal of the quality of quality-of-life measurements. *JAMA: Journal of the American Medical Association* 272(8):619–26.

Guyatt G H, Cook D J 1994 Health status, quality of life, and the individual. *JAMA: Journal of the American Medical Association* 272(8):630–1.

Guyatt G H, Feeny D H, Patrick D L 1993 Measuring health-related quality of life. *Annals of Internal Medicine* 118(8):622–9.

Haas B K 1999 Clarification and integration of similar quality of life concepts. *Image: Journal of Nursing Scholarship* 31(3):215–20.

Heller R F, Knapp J, Valenti L, Dobson A 1993 Secondary prevention after acute myocardial infarction. *American Journal of Cardiology* 72:759–62.

Hillers T K, Guyatt G H, Oldridge N et al 1994 Quality of life after myocardial infarction. *Journal of Clinical Epidemiology* 47(11):1287–96.

Hunt S M, McEwan J, McKenna S P 1986 *Measuring health status.* Croom Helm, London.

Hunt S M, McKenna S P, McEwen J et al 1981 The Nottingham Health Profile: subjective health status and medical consultations. *Social Science and Medicine* 15:221–9.

Katz D A, McHorney C A 2002 The relationship between insomnia and health-related quality of life in patients with chronic illness. *Journal of Family Practice* 51(3):229–35.

Katz S, Ford A, Moskowitz R et al 1963 Studies of illness in the aged. The index of ADL: a standardized measure of biological and psychosocial function. *Journal of the American Medical Association* 185:914–19.

Knobel H, Loge J, Brenne E et al 2003 The validity of EORTC QLQ–C30 fatigue scale in advanced cancer patients and cancer survivors. *Palliative Medicine* 17(8):664–72.

Lawton M P 1971 The functional assessment of elderly people. *Journal of the American Geriatric Society* 19:465–81.

Lim L L-Y, Johnson N A, O'Connell R L, Heller R F 1998 Quality of life and later adverse health outcomes in patients with suspected heart attack. *Australian and New Zealand Journal of Public Health* 22(5):540–6.

Lim L L-Y, Valenti L A, Knapp J C et al 1993 A self-administered quality-of-life questionnaire after acute myocardial infarction. *Journal of Clinical Epidemiology* 46(11):1249–56.

Litaker D, Mion L, Planavsky L et al 2003 Physician–nurse practitioner teams in chronic disease management: the impact on costs, clinical effectiveness, and patients' perception of care. *Journal of Interprofessional Care* 17(3):223–38.

Mayou R, Bryant B 1993 Quality of life in cardiovascular disease. *British Heart Journal* 69:460–6.

McDowell J K 1995 Social support, burden, and psychiatric symptomatology in caregivers: a comparative study, Honours thesis, Queensland University of Technology.

McDowell I, Newell C 1996 *Measuring health. A guide to rating scales and questionnaires*, 2nd edn. Oxford University Press, New York.

Murphy D A, Marelich W D, Dello Stritto M E et al 2002 Mothers living with HIV/AIDS: mental, physical, and family functioning. *AIDS Care* 14(5):633–44.

Oldridge N B 1997 Outcome assessment in cardiac rehabilitation: health-related quality of life and economic evaluation. *Journal of Cardiopulmonary Rehabilitation* 17:179–94.

Oldridge N, Gottlieb M, Guyatt G et al 1998 Predictors of health-related quality of life with cardiac rehabilitation after acute myocardial infarction. *Journal of Cardiopulmonary Rehabilitation* 18(2):95–103.

Oldridge N, Guyatt G, Jones N et al 1991 Effects on quality of life with comprehensive rehabilitation after acute myocardial infarction. *The American Journal of Cardiology* 67:1084–9.

Patrick D L, Erickson P 1993 Assessing health-related quality of life for clinical decision-making, in S R Walker & R M Rosser (eds), *Quality of life assessment: key issues in the 1990s*, pp 11–63. Kluwer Academic Publishers, Dordrecht.

Reinhardt J P, Boerner K, Benn D 2003 Predicting individual change in support over time among chronically impaired older adults, *Psychology and Aging* 18(4):770–9.

Rumsfeld J S, MaWhinney S, McCarthy M et al 1999 Health-related quality of life as a predictor of mortality following coronary artery bypass graft surgery. *JAMA: Journal of the American Medical Association* 281(14):1298–303.

Salek S 1998 *Compendium of quality of life instruments*. John Wiley & Sons, Chichester.

Sanders C, Egger M, Donovan J et al 1998 Reporting on quality of life in randomised controlled trials: bibliographic study. *British Medical Journal* 317:1191–4.

Sharp L K, Lipsky M S 2002 Screening for depression across the lifespan: a review of measures for use in primary care settings. *American Family Physician* 66(6):1001–9.

Slavin L A, Compas B E 1989 The problem of confounding social support and depressive symptoms: a brief report on a college sample. *American Journal of Community Psychology* 17(1):57–66.

Smith H J, Taylor R, Mitchell A 2000 A comparison of four quality of life instruments in cardiac patients: SF–36, QLI, QLMI, and SEIQoL. *Heart* 84:390–4.

Spertus J A, Winder J A, Dewhurst T A et al 1995 Development and evaluation of the Seattle Angina Questionnaire: a new functional status measure for coronary artery disease. *Journal of the American College of Cardiology* 25(2):333–41.

Valenti L, Lim L, Heller R F, Knapp J 1996 An improved questionnaire for assessing quality of life after acute myocardial infarction. *Quality of Life Research* 5(1):151–61.

Walker S R, Rosser R M (eds) 1993 *Quality of life assessment: key issues in the 1990s*. Kluwer Academic Publishers, Dordrecht.

Ware J E, Kosinski M, Keller S D 1994 *SF–36 Physical and Mental Health Summary Scales: a user's manual*. The Health Institute, New England Medical Center, Boston, Massachusetts.

Ware J E, Sherbourne C D 1992 The MOS 36-item short-form health survey (SF–36): I. Conceptual framework and item selection. *Medical Care* 30(6):473–83.

Ware J E, Snow K K, Kosinski M, Gandek B 1993 *SF–36 Health Survey: manual and interpretation guide*. The Health Institute, New England Medical Center, Boston, Massachusetts.

Wenger N K, Mattson M E, Furberg C D, Elinson J 1984 Overview: assessment of quality of life in clinical trials of cardiovascular therapies, in N K Wenger, M E Mattson, C D Furberg & J Elinson (eds), *Assessment of quality of life in clinical trials of cardiovascular therapies*. Le Jacq Publishing Company, New York.

Wright L K, Litaker M, Laraia M, DeAndrade S 2001 Continuum of care for Alzheimer's disease: a nurse education and counselling program. *Issues in Mental Health Nursing* 22(3):231–52.

Zarit S H, Femia E E, Gatz M, Johansson B 1999 Prevalence, incidence and correlates of depression in the oldest old: the OCTO study. *Aging & Mental Health* 3(2):119–28.

index ————————●